MY BOOK

MASON PREDDY

MASON MAISON
PUBLISHING™
REWRITING THE NARRATIVE
MASONMAISON.PUB

MASON MAISON
PUBLISHING™
REWRITING THE NARRATIVE
MASONMAISON.PUB

Copyright & Disclaimer — Pharmacist

This content is provided for educational and informational purposes only and does not constitute medical, legal, or professional advice. The roles, technologies, and clinical processes described represent general best practices that may vary by institution or licensure. Readers should always consult qualified mentors, supervisors, and regulatory sources before making clinical or career decisions.

All names, patient details, and identifying circumstances have been changed or fictionalized to protect privacy. References to Hopewell Hospital for Tomorrow and related entities are part of the creative educational universe of What Color Are Your Scrubs?.

Pharmacists, pharmacy technicians, and students are invited to use this section as a learning companion — an opportunity to explore alignment, stewardship, and safety in the practice of pharmacy. Always follow institutional policies, national standards, and the guidance of licensed professionals.

MASONMAISON.PUB

Printed in the United States of America

Precision is their language, compassion their purpose. Pharmacists stand at the intersection of science and safety—translating chemistry into care, and vigilance into trust. Every label, every dose, every quiet double-check is a silent promise: someone's tomorrow will be safer because of today's accuracy.

1

WELCOME

Introduction — Why Pharmacy Matters

Pharmacy is often described as the science of medications, but the heart of the profession is people. Every dose represents a decision, every label a promise, and every counseling moment a bridge between fear and understanding. Pharmacists stand where chemistry meets compassion, translating complex evidence into everyday safety for the patients and families who trust them.

This section was created to answer the questions students, career-changers, and new clinicians ask most—without sugarcoating the realities or dimming the hope. You'll find practical insight on training, licensure, career paths, and the technology reshaping the profession, alongside the human skills that make the difference when stakes are high. Think of it as a mentor in print: honest, specific, and on your side.

As you move through the Q&A, notice how often the themes repeat: accuracy as compassion, collaboration as strength, and curiosity as a career strategy. If one answer could summarize the rest, it would be this—pharmacy is about protecting life through knowledge. The deeper you go, the more you'll discover that the real measure of expertise is how safely, clearly, and respectfully you help others heal.

Wherever you're starting—from pre-reqs to PGY-2, from retail to research—there's a path here with your name on it. Use these questions to clarify your goals, build your skills, and design a sustainable, meaningful career. And remember: the most important tool you carry isn't in a drawer; it's your judgment, shaped by humility and practice.

2

THE 202™ ABOUT A PHARMACY CAREER + BONUS!

1. What does a pharmacist actually do?

Pharmacists are the bridge between medicine and patient safety. They ensure that every drug dispensed is appropriate, effective, and safe for the individual receiving it. Beyond checking prescriptions, they collaborate with healthcare teams, counsel patients, and monitor therapies to prevent harm while promoting healing. Their role requires both scientific precision and human understanding, as every decision impacts a real person. Over time, the work becomes less about dispensing and more about accountability, where each verification carries meaningful responsibility.

2. Is pharmacy more clinical or retail?

Pharmacy is both, and that duality defines the profession. Clinical pharmacists work directly with providers in hospitals and clinics, while retail pharmacists serve as highly accessible healthcare professionals in the community. The core responsibility remains the same across both settings—ensuring safe and appropriate medication use. However, the pace, workflow, and type of interaction vary significantly. Understanding which environment fits your personality is one of the most important early decisions you will make.

3. What's the difference between a pharmacist and a pharmacy technician?

Pharmacy technicians support the operational side of medication preparation, while pharmacists carry the full clinical and legal responsibility. Technicians manage tasks like filling, labeling, and inventory, allowing pharmacists to focus on verification and patient care. This division of labor improves efficiency and safety. A strong working relationship between the two roles is essential for smooth workflow. Ultimately, the pharmacist is responsible for the final decision and patient outcome.

4. What degree do you need?

To become a pharmacist in the United States, you need a Doctor of Pharmacy (PharmD) from an accredited program. This typically requires completing prerequisite undergraduate coursework followed by four years of pharmacy school. The curriculum includes science, clinical training, and patient interaction. Students learn both technical knowledge and communication skills. By graduation, the expectation is readiness for real-world decision-making.

5. Is a residency required?

A residency is not required for all pharmacists, but it is often expected for clinical roles. These programs provide advanced training and hands-on experience in patient care settings. They help bridge the gap between academic knowledge and real-world practice. While they delay full earning potential, they expand long-term opportunities. The decision should be based on your career goals and desired work environment.

. . .

6. What does a clinical pharmacist do?

Clinical pharmacists are part of the healthcare team, focusing on medication optimization and patient safety. They review lab results, assess therapies, and collaborate with providers to improve outcomes. Their role often includes adjusting medications and preventing adverse effects. Much of their work happens behind the scenes. Despite limited visibility, their impact is significant.

7. What kind of science background is needed?

Pharmacy requires a strong foundation in biology, chemistry, and physiology. Understanding drug interactions and body systems is essential. Students must move beyond memorization to critical thinking. Math and data interpretation also play a role in dosing and safety. This scientific base supports every clinical decision.

8. Do pharmacists prescribe medications?

In some settings, pharmacists have limited prescribing authority under specific protocols. These include areas like immunizations and chronic condition management. Even without direct prescribing, pharmacists influence most medication decisions. Their recommendations guide therapy adjustments. The role is evolving toward greater clinical involvement.

9. What's the difference between a PharmD and a PhD in pharmacy?

A PharmD focuses on patient care, while a PhD focuses on research. PharmDs work directly with patients and healthcare teams. PhDs conduct research and develop new therapies. Both contribute to healthcare in different ways. The choice depends on your interests and career goals.

. . .

10. Can pharmacists specialize?

Yes, pharmacists can specialize in areas like oncology, cardiology, and infectious disease. Specialization often requires additional training or certification. It allows deeper expertise and more complex patient care. These roles can be highly rewarding. They also require continued learning and commitment.

11. How long does it take to become a pharmacist?

Becoming a pharmacist typically takes six to eight years. This includes undergraduate coursework and a PharmD program. Some accelerated programs exist but are still intensive. The timeline reflects the complexity of the role. It is a long-term commitment.

12. What GPA is needed for pharmacy school?

Most programs require at least a 3.0 GPA, though higher is competitive. Science courses carry the most weight. Admissions also consider experience and communication skills. Strong grades alone are not enough. Programs look for well-rounded candidates.

13. Do I need the PCAT?

Many schools no longer require the PCAT. Admissions now focus more on holistic evaluation. Some students still take it to strengthen their application. Requirements vary by program. It is best to research each school individually.

14. What kind of internships are available?

Pharmacy students complete experiential rotations known as IPPEs and APPEs. These provide real-world exposure in different settings. Internships help develop clinical judgment and communication. They connect classroom learning to patient care. Experience gained here is critical.

. . .

15. How do residencies work?

Residencies are structured postgraduate training programs. PGY1 focuses on general clinical practice, while PGY2 adds specialization. Residents work under experienced pharmacists. They gain hands-on experience and develop expertise. These programs open doors to advanced roles.

16. Is pharmacy school difficult?

Pharmacy school is challenging and demanding. It requires strong time management and discipline. The material is complex and fast-paced. Success depends on consistency and effort. Most graduates find it rewarding despite the difficulty.

17. Can I work during pharmacy school?

Many students work as pharmacy interns while in school. This provides both income and practical experience. Balancing work and study requires discipline. It can enhance understanding of coursework. It also helps clarify career direction.

18. What soft skills matter most?

Communication, empathy, and critical thinking are essential. Pharmacists must explain complex information clearly. Emotional intelligence helps with patient interactions. Teamwork is also important in healthcare settings. These skills support both safety and effectiveness.

19. How do students gain patient-care experience?

Students gain experience through rotations and internships. They interact with real patients under supervision. These experiences build confidence and competence. They also improve communication skills. Patient care becomes more intuitive over time.

20. Do pharmacists take board exams?

Yes, pharmacists must pass licensure exams. The NAPLEX tests clinical knowledge. The MPJE covers pharmacy law. Some states have additional requirements. These exams ensure readiness for practice.

21. What are common pharmacist career paths?

Pharmacists can work in retail, hospital, clinical, industry, or academia. Each path offers different experiences and challenges. Some focus on patient interaction, others on research or systems. The profession offers flexibility. Career paths can evolve over time.

22. What does a retail pharmacist do?

Retail pharmacists fill prescriptions and counsel patients. They also administer vaccines and provide health screenings. The role involves high volume and constant interaction. Customer service is a major component. It blends clinical knowledge with accessibility.

23. What is a hospital pharmacist's day like?

Hospital pharmacists review orders and collaborate with care teams. They monitor patient therapies and adjust medications. Their work is more clinical and less customer-facing. The pace can vary depending on the unit. Their impact is critical to patient safety.

24. Can pharmacists work in research?

Yes, pharmacists can work in research settings. They design studies and analyze data. Research roles focus on discovery and innovation. These positions are less patient-facing. They contribute to advancing medicine.

25. What is an ambulatory care pharmacist?

Ambulatory care pharmacists work in outpatient settings. They manage chronic conditions and adjust therapies. They often build long-term patient relationships. Their work focuses on continuity of care. This role is growing in demand.

Section 3 — Career Pathways (Q26–50)

26. What is a clinical pharmacy specialist?

A clinical pharmacy specialist is a pharmacist with advanced training in a specific area of care. They often complete residencies and obtain board certifications. These pharmacists work closely with physicians and manage complex patient cases. Their role includes making therapy recommendations and monitoring outcomes. They are considered subject-matter experts within their specialty.

27. What is a compounding pharmacist?

Compounding pharmacists create customized medications for individual patients. This may include altering dosage forms or removing allergens. They work in specialized pharmacies that follow strict preparation standards. Accuracy and sterility are critical in this role. It requires both technical skill and attention to detail.

28. What is a pharmaceutical industry pharmacist?

Pharmacists in the pharmaceutical industry work in areas like research, medical affairs, and drug safety. They may help develop new medications or educate providers about existing ones. These roles often involve less direct patient interaction. The focus shifts from individual patients to broader populations. It is a different application of the same knowledge base.

29. What is a managed care pharmacist?

Managed care pharmacists work with insurance companies and healthcare systems. They help determine which medications are covered and how they are used. Their work focuses on cost-effectiveness and population health. They analyze data and develop policies. This role blends clinical knowledge with systems thinking.

30. What is a consultant pharmacist?

Consultant pharmacists provide medication expertise in settings like nursing homes and long-term care facilities. They review medication regimens and ensure safety for vulnerable populations. Their role includes identifying unnecessary or harmful medications. They often work independently or with limited supervision. This role emphasizes oversight and optimization.

31. Can pharmacists work in academia?

Yes, pharmacists can become professors or educators. They teach students and may also conduct research. Academic roles combine instruction with scholarship. Many also maintain clinical practice. This path requires strong communication and subject mastery.

32. What is an infectious disease pharmacist?

Infectious disease pharmacists specialize in treating infections. They focus on antibiotic use and resistance. Their role is critical in preventing misuse of medications. They often work in hospitals and collaborate with physicians. Their decisions impact both individual patients and public health.

. . .

33. What is an oncology pharmacist?

Oncology pharmacists work with cancer patients and chemotherapy treatments. They ensure medications are dosed correctly and safely. This role carries high responsibility due to the risk involved. Emotional resilience is important in this setting. Their work directly affects patient outcomes in critical situations.

34. What is a critical care pharmacist?

Critical care pharmacists work in intensive care units. They manage medications for severely ill patients. Their environment is fast-paced and high-stakes. They must make decisions quickly and accurately. Their role is essential in emergency and life-threatening situations.

35. What is a pediatric pharmacist?

Pediatric pharmacists specialize in treating children. Dosing is often weight-based and requires precision. They must consider developmental differences in patients. Communication with families is also important. This role requires both accuracy and empathy.

36. Can pharmacists work remotely?

Yes, some pharmacists work in telepharmacy or remote verification roles. These positions allow them to review prescriptions and provide consultations from a distance. Technology enables these opportunities. However, not all roles can be performed remotely. The availability depends on the setting.

37. What is telepharmacy?

Telepharmacy involves providing pharmacy services through technology. Pharmacists verify medications and consult patients remotely. It improves access in underserved areas. Communication skills are essential in this format. It is a growing part of the profession.

38. What is a medication safety pharmacist?

Medication safety pharmacists focus on preventing errors. They analyze incidents and improve systems. Their work involves policy development and staff education. They aim to reduce risk across the organization. This role is proactive rather than reactive.

39. What is a regulatory pharmacist?

Regulatory pharmacists work with government agencies or companies. They ensure medications meet safety and compliance standards. Their work involves reviewing data and documentation. They help bring drugs to market safely. This role requires strong attention to detail.

40. Can pharmacists start their own business?

Yes, pharmacists can own independent pharmacies or consulting businesses. Entrepreneurship offers autonomy and flexibility. However, it also involves financial risk and management responsibilities. Business skills become as important as clinical knowledge. Success depends on both areas.

41. What are the most flexible pharmacy careers?

Some pharmacy roles offer more flexibility than others. Remote positions, consulting, and per diem work provide more control over schedules. Retail and hospital roles are typically more structured. Flexibility often comes with experience. It requires planning and positioning.

. . .

42. What are the highest-paying pharmacy jobs?

Pharmaceutical industry roles often offer the highest salaries. Specialized clinical positions and leadership roles also pay well. Compensation varies by location and experience. Higher pay usually comes with increased responsibility. It is important to balance income with alignment.

43. What pharmacy roles involve the most patient interaction?

Retail and ambulatory care pharmacists have the most direct patient contact. These roles involve counseling and ongoing communication. Hospital pharmacists typically have less interaction. The level of patient contact varies by setting. Choosing the right environment matters.

44. What pharmacy roles involve the least patient interaction?

Industry, informatics, and regulatory roles involve less direct patient contact. These positions focus on systems, data, or research. They appeal to those who prefer behind-the-scenes work. The impact is still significant but less visible. These roles offer a different type of fulfillment.

45. Can pharmacists transition between roles?

Yes, pharmacists can move between different career paths. Transitions may require additional training or experience. Networking and planning make the process easier. Early decisions can influence flexibility later. It is possible but not always immediate.

46. What is pharmacy informatics?

Pharmacy informatics focuses on technology and data systems. Pharmacists in this field improve workflows and medication safety through systems. They work with electronic health records and analytics tools. This role blends clinical knowledge with IT skills. It is a growing area.

47. What is pharmacovigilance?

Pharmacovigilance involves monitoring drug safety after approval. Pharmacists track adverse events and ensure proper reporting. This work helps protect patients on a large scale. It is often done in industry or regulatory settings. The focus is on long-term safety.

48. What is a nuclear pharmacist?

Nuclear pharmacists prepare radioactive medications for diagnostic imaging and treatment. This role requires specialized training and certification. Precision and safety are critical due to radiation exposure. Work environments are controlled and highly regulated. It is a niche but important field.

49. What is a specialty pharmacist?

Specialty pharmacists manage complex and high-cost medications. These often treat chronic or rare conditions. They coordinate care, insurance, and patient education. Their role involves close monitoring and follow-up. This field is rapidly growing.

50. What is the most stable pharmacy career path?

Many pharmacy careers offer stability due to consistent demand. Retail and hospital roles are generally reliable. Stability depends on location and market trends. Some specialized roles may be more competitive. Long-term stability comes from adaptability and alignment.

Section 6 — Pay, Demand & Outlook / Section 7 — Specializations / Section 8 — Ethics & Law (Q51–75)

. . .

51. How much do pharmacists make?

Pharmacist salaries vary by setting, location, and experience. Many pharmacists earn a six-figure income, especially in retail and hospital roles. Industry and specialized positions may offer higher earning potential. Compensation often reflects responsibility and workload. Salary should be considered alongside job satisfaction and long-term sustainability.

52. Does location affect pharmacist salary?

Yes, geographic location plays a significant role in salary. Urban areas may offer higher pay but also come with higher cost of living. Rural areas sometimes offer incentives to attract pharmacists. Regional demand can influence compensation packages. It is important to evaluate both income and lifestyle when considering location.

53. Is pharmacy a growing field?

Pharmacy continues to evolve as healthcare changes. Some areas show growth, especially in specialty and clinical roles. However, other areas may feel saturated depending on location. Demand is not evenly distributed across the profession. Understanding where growth is happening is key.

54. Is there a pharmacist shortage?

The idea of a shortage depends on the setting. Some retail environments experience high turnover and ongoing demand. Clinical roles can be competitive due to training requirements. The issue is often misalignment rather than pure shortage. Workforce trends vary widely.

55. What affects job availability?

Job availability is influenced by location, experience, and specialization. Residency training can impact access to certain roles. Market saturation in specific regions also plays a role. Employers may seek candidates with prior experience. Strategic planning improves opportunities.

56. How competitive are clinical pharmacy jobs?

Clinical roles are often more competitive than retail positions. Many require residency training or specialized experience. Applicants may need strong academic and clinical backgrounds. Networking can also influence opportunities. Preparation is important for entering this path.

57. Is pharmacy financially worth it?

Pharmacy can offer a stable and strong income over time. However, the cost of education and student debt must be considered. Financial outcomes depend on career choices and repayment strategies. Long-term planning is essential. The decision should align with both financial and personal goals.

58. What is the job outlook for pharmacists?

The job outlook varies by role and location. Some traditional roles may see slower growth. New opportunities are emerging in clinical and specialty areas. Technology is also influencing the profession. Adaptability will shape long-term success.

59. How does debt impact pharmacists?

Many pharmacists graduate with significant student loan debt. This can influence career choices and financial decisions. Repayment strategies vary widely. Debt may delay certain life goals. Understanding this reality is important before committing.

. . .

60. Can pharmacists achieve financial independence?

Yes, many pharmacists can achieve financial stability and independence. This depends on income, spending, and debt management. Career choices also influence earning potential. Planning and discipline are key factors. Financial success is possible with intention.

61. What are the most popular pharmacy specialties?

Common specialties include oncology, cardiology, and infectious disease. These areas require additional training and certification. They offer opportunities for advanced practice. Specialization allows deeper expertise. It also shapes long-term career direction.

62. How do pharmacists choose a specialty?

Choosing a specialty often depends on interests and experiences during training. Exposure through rotations helps clarify preferences. Mentorship can guide decisions. Some specialties require residency training. Alignment with personality is important.

63. What is ambulatory care pharmacy?

Ambulatory care pharmacists work with patients in outpatient settings. They manage chronic conditions and adjust therapies. These roles often involve direct patient interaction. Continuity of care is a key focus. This area is growing in demand.

64. What is cardiology pharmacy?

Cardiology pharmacists specialize in heart-related conditions. They manage medications for diseases like hypertension and heart failure. Their role requires detailed knowledge of cardiovascular drugs. They often work in hospitals or clinics. Their decisions impact long-term patient health.

. . .

65. What is oncology pharmacy?

Oncology pharmacists focus on cancer treatment medications. They ensure proper dosing and monitor for side effects. The work requires precision and emotional resilience. These roles are highly specialized. Patient safety is critical in this field.

66. What is infectious disease pharmacy?

Infectious disease pharmacists manage antibiotic use and treatment plans. They play a key role in preventing resistance. Their work supports both individual patients and public health. They often collaborate with healthcare teams. This specialty requires strong clinical knowledge.

67. What is psychiatric pharmacy?

Psychiatric pharmacists specialize in mental health medications. They help manage conditions like depression and anxiety. Their role involves careful monitoring and adjustments. Communication with patients is essential. This field requires empathy and patience.

68. What is pediatric pharmacy?

Pediatric pharmacists work with children and infants. Dosing is often based on weight and requires precision. They consider developmental differences in patients. Their role involves both safety and communication. This specialty requires careful attention.

69. What is geriatric pharmacy?

Geriatric pharmacists focus on elderly patients. They manage multiple medications and reduce risks. Their role includes simplifying regimens and preventing interactions. They work in various healthcare settings. This specialty supports aging populations.

. . .

70. What is critical care pharmacy?

Critical care pharmacists work in intensive care environments. They manage medications for severely ill patients. The pace is fast and the stakes are high. Decisions must be made quickly and accurately. This role requires confidence and expertise.

71. What ethical responsibilities do pharmacists have?

Pharmacists are responsible for patient safety and confidentiality. They must act in the best interest of patients. Ethical decisions are part of daily practice. Integrity is essential in this role. Trust is built through consistent behavior.

72. What is patient confidentiality in pharmacy?

Patient confidentiality involves protecting personal health information. Pharmacists must follow strict privacy laws. This includes secure handling of records. Violations can have serious consequences. Maintaining trust is critical.

73. What is informed consent?

Informed consent means patients understand their treatment. Pharmacists help explain medications and risks. Patients must be able to make informed decisions. Communication plays a key role. This supports patient autonomy.

74. What happens if a pharmacist makes an error?

Errors are taken seriously and must be addressed. Pharmacists report and analyze mistakes. The goal is to prevent future occurrences. Systems are often improved as a result. Accountability is part of the profession.

. . .

75. How do pharmacists handle ethical dilemmas?

Pharmacists rely on professional guidelines and judgment. They consider patient safety and legal requirements. Consultation with colleagues may be necessary. Ethical decisions can be complex. Experience helps guide these situations.

Section 8–10 — Ethics, Technology, Purpose & Reflection (Q76–101)

76. What is professional integrity in pharmacy?

Professional integrity means consistently doing the right thing, even when it's difficult or unnoticed. Pharmacists must make decisions that prioritize patient safety over convenience or pressure. This includes being honest about uncertainties and correcting mistakes when they occur. Integrity builds trust with both patients and healthcare teams. Over time, it becomes one of the most important qualities in the profession.

77. How do pharmacists handle conflicts with providers?

Pharmacists may sometimes disagree with prescribing providers. These situations require respectful communication and clinical reasoning. The goal is always patient safety, not proving a point. Strong relationships make these conversations easier. Confidence and professionalism are key.

78. What legal responsibilities do pharmacists have?

Pharmacists are legally responsible for the medications they dispense. They must follow federal and state laws. This includes proper documentation and verification. Errors can have legal consequences. Understanding regulations is essential for safe practice.

79. What is medication error reporting?

Medication error reporting involves documenting mistakes or near misses. This helps identify patterns and improve systems. The goal is learning, not punishment. Reporting improves patient safety over time. Transparency is essential.

80. Why is ethics important in pharmacy?

Ethics guide decision-making in complex situations. Pharmacists must balance clinical knowledge with patient needs. Ethical practice ensures trust and safety. It supports professional standards. Without ethics, safe care is not possible.

81. How is technology changing pharmacy?

Technology is transforming how pharmacists work. Electronic systems manage prescriptions and patient data. Automation improves efficiency and accuracy. However, it also increases reliance on digital tools. Pharmacists must adapt to these changes.

82. What is an electronic health record (EHR)?

An EHR is a digital version of a patient's medical history. Pharmacists use it to review medications and lab results. It improves communication across healthcare teams. Access to accurate information supports better decisions. EHR systems are central to modern practice.

83. What is clinical decision support?

Clinical decision support systems provide alerts and recommendations. They help identify drug interactions and dosing issues. These tools improve safety but are not perfect. Pharmacists must interpret alerts carefully. Judgment remains essential.

. . .

84. What is automation in pharmacy?

Automation includes machines that prepare and dispense medications. It improves efficiency and reduces manual errors. Pharmacists oversee these systems rather than replace them. This shifts focus toward clinical tasks. Technology supports—but does not replace—expertise.

85. What is telepharmacy's future?

Telepharmacy is expected to grow in the coming years. It expands access to care in underserved areas. Pharmacists can work remotely and provide consultations. Technology makes this possible. It adds flexibility to the profession.

86. Will AI replace pharmacists?

AI will assist pharmacists but not replace them. It can analyze data and identify patterns quickly. However, human judgment is still necessary for decision-making. Patient care requires context and communication. Pharmacists remain essential.

87. How do pharmacists stay current?

Pharmacists complete continuing education regularly. They attend conferences and review new research. Staying current is required for licensure. It ensures safe and effective practice. Lifelong learning is part of the profession.

88. What role does data play in pharmacy?

Data helps pharmacists make informed decisions. It includes patient history, lab results, and medication records. Analyzing data improves outcomes and safety. Pharmacists must interpret information accurately. Data-driven care is becoming more important.

. . .

89. What is digital fatigue in pharmacy?

Digital fatigue comes from constant interaction with systems and screens. Pharmacists manage multiple alerts and data sources. This can lead to mental exhaustion. It requires focus and discipline to manage. Recognizing it is the first step to addressing it.

90. How does technology affect workload?

Technology can both reduce and increase workload. It improves efficiency but adds new tasks. Alerts and documentation can become overwhelming. Pharmacists must manage this balance. Workflow awareness is critical.

91. What gives pharmacists a sense of purpose?

Purpose often comes from knowing their work protects patients. Even small interventions can prevent harm. The impact may not always be visible. Many pharmacists find meaning in consistency and reliability. Purpose is often quiet but powerful.

92. How do pharmacists measure success?

Success is not always measured by recognition. It is often defined by safe outcomes and avoided errors. Consistency and accuracy matter most. Personal satisfaction may come from small wins. Success looks different over time.

93. What keeps pharmacists motivated?

Motivation varies from person to person. Some are driven by patient impact, others by problem-solving. A supportive environment can make a difference. Growth opportunities also help sustain motivation. Alignment plays a key role.

. . .

94. What challenges long-term satisfaction?

Burnout, workload, and misalignment can affect satisfaction. Repetitive tasks may feel draining over time. Lack of recognition can also be a factor. Environment matters as much as the role itself. Addressing these early helps long-term success.

95. What does burnout look like in pharmacy?

Burnout often appears as mental fatigue and disengagement. It builds gradually rather than suddenly. Pharmacists may feel less connected to their work. Irritation and exhaustion can increase. Recognizing it early is important.

96. How can pharmacists maintain balance?

Maintaining balance requires boundaries and self-awareness. Time management and workload control are important. Support systems also help. Balance is not automatic—it must be created. Long-term sustainability depends on it.

97. What role does alignment play in career satisfaction?

Alignment determines whether the work fits the individual. It includes personality, environment, and expectations. When alignment is strong, work feels sustainable. When it is weak, burnout increases. Alignment is more important than capability.

98. How do pharmacists grow over time?

Growth comes through experience and continued learning. Pharmacists develop confidence and efficiency. They may specialize or change roles. Reflection helps guide decisions. Growth is both professional and personal.

. . .

99. What is the biggest lesson pharmacists learn?

Many pharmacists learn that responsibility defines the role. It is not just about medications. Every decision carries weight. This realization shapes their approach to work. It becomes central to their identity.

100. What should I think about before choosing pharmacy?

You should consider both the rewards and challenges. Understanding the day-to-day reality is critical. Financial and lifestyle factors also matter. Talking to practicing pharmacists can provide insight. A well-informed decision leads to better outcomes.

101. If I'm being completely honest with myself, should I become a Clinical Pharmacist — or would another path fit me better?

This question is about alignment, not ability. Becoming a Clinical Pharmacist requires sustained focus, precision, and responsibility. The role often involves high impact with limited visibility. Some people find this deeply fulfilling, while others find it draining. The right answer depends on whether the work fits how you think, operate, and want to live over time.

102. What is the hardest part of being a Clinical Pharmacist that people don't talk about?

The hardest part is the constant responsibility that never fully turns off. Even when your shift ends, the weight of decisions can linger in the back of your mind. You may find yourself replaying orders, questioning whether something could have been done differently. It's not anxiety—it's accountability. Learning how to carry that weight without letting it consume you is one of the most important skills in the profession.

103. Do Clinical Pharmacists ever feel unsure about their decisions?

Yes, and that's actually a sign of a thoughtful practitioner. Medicine is rarely black and white, and even experienced pharmacists encounter gray areas. The key is not eliminating uncertainty, but managing it through evidence, collaboration, and experience. Over time, confidence grows—but humility should remain. The best pharmacists question just enough to stay sharp.

104. How do you handle making a mistake in pharmacy?

Mistakes are taken seriously, but they are also opportunities to improve systems. The focus is on identifying what happened, why it happened, and how to prevent it from happening again. Transparency is critical—hiding errors creates more risk than the error itself. Most institutions prioritize learning over punishment when issues are reported appropriately. Growth in pharmacy often comes from these difficult moments.

105. Is burnout common in Clinical Pharmacy?

Burnout can occur, especially in high-pressure environments with constant interruptions and workload demands. It often stems from misalignment rather than lack of capability. Pharmacists who are highly detail-oriented may struggle in chaotic settings, while others may feel disengaged in slower roles. Recognizing early signs and adjusting your environment when possible is essential. Sustainability matters more than short-term performance.

106. How important is communication in this role?

Communication is just as important as clinical knowledge. A recommendation is only valuable if it is understood and accepted by the care team. Pharmacists must be able to explain complex concepts clearly and confidently. This includes knowing when to speak up and when to listen. Strong communication builds trust—and trust increases your impact.

107. What kind of mindset helps you succeed as a Clinical Pharmacist?

A mindset focused on curiosity, accountability, and continuous improvement is key. You must be willing to learn constantly, adapt to new information, and refine your approach. Rigid thinking can limit your effectiveness in a field that evolves rapidly. At the same time, consistency and discipline provide stability. The balance between flexibility and structure defines long-term success.

108. Do Clinical Pharmacists work independently or as part of a team?

Both. While much of the work involves independent verification and analysis, collaboration is constant. Pharmacists interact with physicians, nurses, and other healthcare professionals throughout the day. Decisions are often made within a team context, even when the pharmacist's role is advisory. The ability to function in both modes is essential.

109. How do you keep up with new medications and guidelines?

Ongoing education is built into the profession. Pharmacists use clinical databases, journals, continuing education programs, and professional networks to stay current. Learning is not occasional—it is continuous. Many also develop personal systems for tracking updates in their specialty areas. Staying informed is part of the responsibility, not an optional extra.

110. What is the most rewarding part of being a Clinical Pharmacist?

The most rewarding part is knowing that your work directly improves patient safety and outcomes. Often, the impact is invisible—an error prevented, a dose adjusted, a therapy optimized. These moments may not be recognized publicly, but they matter deeply. Over time, those small interventions add up to significant impact. That sense of purpose is what keeps many pharmacists committed to the field.

111. How do Clinical Pharmacists handle disagreement with physicians?

Disagreements are handled professionally and with a focus on patient safety. Pharmacists present evidence, guidelines, and clinical reasoning rather than personal opinion. Most physicians respect well-supported recommendations, especially when delivered clearly and calmly. The goal is not to "win" the conversation, but to reach the safest outcome. Strong working relationships make these moments more productive over time.

112. Do Clinical Pharmacists ever feel overlooked?

Yes, especially in roles where much of the work happens behind the scenes. Many of the most important interventions are never visible to patients or even other staff. This can create a sense of being undervalued if recognition is important to you. Over time, pharmacists learn to find fulfillment in impact rather than visibility. Still, workplace culture plays a major role in how valued the role feels.

113. How repetitive is the work in Clinical Pharmacy?

Some aspects are repetitive, especially verification tasks and common medication checks. However, each patient introduces variation, and clinical scenarios are rarely identical. The balance between repetition and complexity depends heavily on the setting. In high-volume environments, repetition may dominate. In clinical or specialty roles, variation tends to be higher.

114. What is the biggest adjustment for new pharmacists?

The biggest adjustment is transitioning from academic knowledge to real-world decision-making. In school, answers are often clear and structured. In practice, information can be incomplete, and decisions must still be made. This shift requires confidence, adaptability, and the ability to tolerate uncertainty. It's a transition that takes time and experience.

115. How do Clinical Pharmacists prioritize their workload?

Prioritization is based on patient acuity, medication risk, and time sensitivity. High-alert medications and unstable patients come first. Pharmacists constantly reassess priorities as new information arrives. This dynamic decision-making is a core part of the role. Strong organizational skills are essential to manage competing demands effectively.

116. Is multitasking required in this profession?

Yes, but it is more accurate to say that pharmacists manage multiple streams of work rather than true multitasking. They shift attention quickly between tasks while maintaining accuracy. Interruptions are common, and the ability to refocus is critical. Over time, this becomes a learned skill rather than an innate ability. Precision must never be sacrificed for speed.

117. How do Clinical Pharmacists manage interruptions?

Interruptions are managed by maintaining a clear mental checkpoint before shifting tasks. Pharmacists often pause briefly to note where they left off before responding to a new request. This reduces the risk of errors when returning to the original task. Over time, structured habits help maintain accuracy despite frequent disruptions. Interruptions are expected, not avoided.

118. What role does technology play in Clinical Pharmacy?

Technology is central to the role, supporting everything from order verification to clinical decision-making. Electronic health records, drug databases, and automated systems enhance efficiency and safety. However, technology is not a replacement for clinical judgment. Pharmacists must interpret and validate information rather than rely on it blindly. The combination of technology and expertise drives optimal outcomes.

119. How important is attention to detail?

Attention to detail is critical and non-negotiable in pharmacy practice. Small errors can have significant consequences, especially with dosing and drug interactions. Pharmacists develop habits that reinforce accuracy, such as double-checking calculations and verifying assumptions. This level of focus must be sustained throughout the shift. Precision is a defining characteristic of the profession.

120. Do Clinical Pharmacists specialize, or are they generalists?

Both paths exist, depending on training and career choices. Some pharmacists remain generalists, working across a broad range of medications and conditions. Others pursue specialized roles in areas like oncology, critical care, or infectious disease. Specialization often requires additional training, such as residency or certification. Each path offers different types of challenges and rewards.

121. How does experience change the role over time?

Experience increases confidence, efficiency, and clinical intuition. Pharmacists become faster at identifying issues and more comfortable making decisions. They also develop stronger communication skills and professional relationships. Over time, the role often expands to include teaching, leadership, or system-level contributions. Experience transforms the job from reactive to proactive.

122. What is the learning curve like for new pharmacists?

The learning curve is steep in the first year, especially in clinical settings. New pharmacists must apply knowledge quickly while adapting to workflow and systems. Mistakes or near-misses can feel intense early on, but they contribute to growth. Support from colleagues and structured onboarding programs can make a significant difference. With time, the curve levels out into confidence.

123. How do Clinical Pharmacists stay organized?

Organization is maintained through structured workflows, checklists, and personal systems. Many pharmacists develop routines for reviewing orders, documenting notes, and tracking tasks. Electronic systems also help manage information, but personal discipline remains key. Staying organized reduces stress and improves accuracy. It is a skill that develops with practice.

124. What is the role of intuition in pharmacy?

Intuition plays a role, but it is built on experience and pattern recognition. Experienced pharmacists often sense when something "doesn't look right" before identifying the exact issue. This instinct complements, but does not replace, evidence-based decision-making. Intuition becomes more reliable over time. It is a product of repeated exposure to clinical scenarios.

125. How do Clinical Pharmacists handle high-pressure situations?

High-pressure situations are managed through preparation, training, and controlled responses. Pharmacists rely on established protocols and clinical knowledge to guide decisions. Staying calm allows for clearer thinking and better outcomes. Over time, exposure to pressure builds resilience. The ability to function under stress is essential in many pharmacy roles.

126. What is the difference between retail and clinical pharmacy experiences?

Retail pharmacy focuses more on volume, patient interaction, and operational efficiency. Clinical pharmacy emphasizes direct involvement in patient care and decision-making within a healthcare team. The pace, responsibilities, and stressors differ significantly between the two. Each environment requires different strengths and preferences. Understanding these differences helps guide career choices.

127. How does collaboration improve patient outcomes?

Collaboration allows multiple perspectives to inform patient care decisions. Pharmacists contribute medication expertise, while physicians and nurses provide additional clinical context. This teamwork reduces errors and improves treatment effectiveness. Open communication is essential for successful collaboration. The combined effort leads to better overall outcomes.

128. What challenges come with working in a team environment?

Challenges include communication gaps, differing opinions, and varying levels of experience. Misalignment within the team can impact workflow and decision-making. Strong interpersonal skills help navigate these challenges effectively. Building trust over time improves collaboration. Successful teams prioritize patient outcomes over individual perspectives.

129. How do Clinical Pharmacists handle difficult conversations?

Difficult conversations are handled with professionalism, clarity, and empathy. Pharmacists focus on facts and patient safety while maintaining respect for others. Listening is as important as speaking in these situations. The goal is to resolve issues constructively rather than create conflict. Strong communication skills are essential.

130. What is the role of leadership in pharmacy?

Leadership can exist at all levels, not just in formal positions. Pharmacists often lead through influence, education, and example. They may guide teams, mentor colleagues, or improve processes. Leadership involves responsibility beyond individual tasks. It shapes both patient care and workplace culture.

131. How do Clinical Pharmacists mentor others?

Mentorship involves sharing knowledge, guiding decision-making, and supporting professional growth. Experienced pharmacists help newer colleagues build confidence and skills. Teaching often occurs informally during daily work. Structured preceptorships provide additional opportunities. Mentorship strengthens both individuals and the profession.

132. What are the most common sources of stress in pharmacy?

Common stressors include workload, time pressure, interruptions, and high responsibility. Emotional factors, such as patient outcomes, also contribute. The specific sources vary by setting and role. Recognizing these stressors helps in managing them effectively. Alignment between the role and personal preferences can reduce long-term stress.

133. How do Clinical Pharmacists manage stress?

Stress is managed through structured routines, support from colleagues, and time away from work. Developing coping strategies is essential for sustainability. Some pharmacists focus on organization and efficiency to reduce stress. Others rely on external activities to reset. There is no single solution, but awareness is key.

134. What is the importance of continuing education?

Continuing education ensures that pharmacists remain current with evolving practices and new medications. It supports safe and effective patient care. Many roles require ongoing certification and training. Learning is continuous in this profession. Staying informed is both a responsibility and an opportunity for growth.

135. How do Clinical Pharmacists adapt to change?

Adaptability is essential due to constant changes in guidelines, medications, and systems. Pharmacists must be willing to learn and adjust quickly. Flexibility helps maintain effectiveness in evolving environments. Resistance to change can limit growth. Successful pharmacists embrace change as part of the role.

136. How do Clinical Pharmacists handle uncertainty in patient care?

Uncertainty is managed by combining available data, clinical guidelines, and professional judgment. Pharmacists rarely have perfect information, so decisions are made based on the best evidence at the time. Collaboration with the care team helps reduce gaps in understanding. Over time, comfort with uncertainty becomes part of the role. The goal is not certainty—it is safe, informed decision-making.

137. What is the role of evidence-based practice in pharmacy?

Evidence-based practice guides clinical decisions using research, guidelines, and proven outcomes. Pharmacists rely on this framework to ensure treatments are both safe and effective. It helps standardize care while allowing for individual patient considerations. Without evidence-based practice, decision-making becomes inconsistent. It is a foundational element of modern pharmacy.

138. How do Clinical Pharmacists balance speed and accuracy?

Balancing speed and accuracy requires discipline and experience. Pharmacists develop workflows that allow them to move efficiently without skipping critical checks. When pressure increases, accuracy must remain the priority. Over time, efficiency improves naturally without sacrificing precision. The balance is learned through repetition and awareness.

139. What is the most common misconception about Clinical Pharmacy?

A common misconception is that pharmacists simply verify medications without deeper involvement. In reality, many clinical pharmacists actively influence treatment decisions. Their role includes identifying risks, optimizing therapy, and collaborating with healthcare teams. The work is far more analytical and impactful than many people realize. Understanding this helps clarify the value of the profession.

140. How do Clinical Pharmacists contribute to patient safety?

They contribute by identifying potential medication errors, interactions, and dosing issues before they reach the patient. Pharmacists act as a final checkpoint in the medication process. Their attention to detail prevents harm that might otherwise go unnoticed. Safety is built through consistent, careful work. This role is one of the most critical contributions pharmacists make.

141. What types of patients do Clinical Pharmacists typically work with?

They work with a wide range of patients, depending on the

setting. This can include critically ill individuals, chronic disease patients, pediatric populations, or specialty cases. Each group presents unique challenges and considerations. The diversity of patients keeps the role dynamic. It also requires adaptability and broad clinical knowledge.

142. How do Clinical Pharmacists support medication adherence?

They educate patients, simplify medication regimens, and address barriers to consistent use. Understanding why a patient is not adhering is key to improving outcomes. Pharmacists may adjust therapy or provide tools to make adherence easier. Communication plays a central role in this process. Long-term success often depends on these efforts.

143. What is the role of documentation in pharmacy practice?

Documentation records clinical decisions, supports continuity of care, and communicates recommendations to the healthcare team. It ensures that actions taken are clear and traceable. Good documentation improves patient outcomes and reduces errors. It also serves as a legal and professional record. Accurate documentation is an essential part of the role.

144. How do Clinical Pharmacists evaluate treatment effectiveness?

They monitor patient outcomes, lab values, and clinical responses to therapy. Adjustments are made based on how well the treatment is working. This process is continuous rather than one-time. Pharmacists use both objective data and clinical observation. Evaluation ensures that therapy remains appropriate over time.

145. What is the importance of teamwork in Clinical Pharmacy?

Teamwork allows for shared decision-making and improved patient outcomes. Each team member contributes a unique perspective. Pharmacists provide medication expertise within this structure. Effective teamwork reduces errors and enhances care quality. Strong collaboration is essential in most pharmacy settings.

146. How do Clinical Pharmacists handle conflicting information?

They evaluate sources critically, prioritize high-quality evidence, and use clinical judgment to resolve discrepancies. Not all information is equally reliable. Pharmacists must determine what is most relevant to the patient. Consultation with colleagues can also help clarify uncertainty. The goal is to make the safest, most informed decision possible.

147. What role does critical thinking play in pharmacy?

Critical thinking allows pharmacists to analyze complex situations and make informed decisions. It goes beyond memorization to understanding how different factors interact. This skill is essential for identifying risks and optimizing therapy. Without critical thinking, errors are more likely. It is one of the most important competencies in the profession.

148. How do Clinical Pharmacists manage time effectively?

Time management involves prioritizing tasks, minimizing distractions, and maintaining structured workflows. Pharmacists often juggle multiple responsibilities simultaneously. Efficient systems help ensure that important tasks are completed on time. Experience improves time management skills. Staying organized reduces stress and improves performance.

149. What is the impact of workload on performance?

High workload can increase the risk of errors if not managed properly. Pharmacists must maintain focus even under pressure. Systems and support structures help mitigate these risks. Awareness of workload limits is important for safety. Maintaining balance is key to long-term effectiveness.

150. How do Clinical Pharmacists ensure accuracy in calculations?

They double-check calculations, use reliable tools, and follow standardized processes. Verification is a routine part of the workflow. Even simple calculations are treated with care. Accuracy is reinforced through habit and discipline. This reduces the likelihood of errors.

151. What is the role of protocols in pharmacy practice?

Protocols provide standardized approaches to common clinical situations. They improve efficiency and reduce variability in care.

Pharmacists use protocols as a guide, not a replacement for judgment. Flexibility is still required for unique cases. Protocols support consistency and safety.

152. How do Clinical Pharmacists stay focused during long shifts?

They use structured workflows, take brief mental resets when possible, and rely on habits to maintain consistency. Fatigue can impact performance, so awareness is important. Small breaks, even brief ones, can help sustain focus. Experience also improves endurance. Maintaining concentration is critical for safety.

153. What is the importance of accuracy in documentation?

Accurate documentation ensures that clinical decisions are clearly communicated and understood. Errors in documentation can lead to incorrect treatment plans. Precision in writing reflects precision in practice. It also supports accountability and continuity. Accuracy is essential at every step.

154. How do Clinical Pharmacists handle complex medication regimens?

They break the regimen into manageable components, evaluate each medication, and assess interactions. Simplifying therapy when possible improves outcomes. Complexity requires careful analysis and planning. Pharmacists use both clinical knowledge and experience. The goal is clarity and safety.

155. What is the role of patient education in pharmacy?

Patient education helps individuals understand their medications and how to use them correctly. It improves adherence and reduces the risk of errors. Pharmacists tailor information to each patient's needs. Clear communication is essential. Education is a key part of patient-centered care.

156. How do Clinical Pharmacists respond to emergencies?

They rely on training, protocols, and experience to act quickly and accurately. Clear communication and calm decision-making are critical. Pharmacists prepare for emergencies through practice and repetition. In high-pressure situations, preparation becomes action. Their role can be vital in stabilizing patients.

157. What is the impact of experience on clinical judgment?

Experience enhances the ability to recognize patterns and make informed decisions quickly. It builds confidence while reinforcing caution. Pharmacists learn from both successes and challenges. Over time, judgment becomes more refined. Experience is one of the most valuable assets in practice.

158. How do Clinical Pharmacists maintain professionalism?

They communicate respectfully, act ethically, and prioritize patient care at all times. Professionalism builds trust within the healthcare team. It also supports effective collaboration. Consistent behavior reinforces credibility. Maintaining professionalism is essential for long-term success.

159. What is the role of ethics in pharmacy practice?

Ethics guide decision-making when situations are complex or unclear. Pharmacists must balance patient needs, safety, and professional responsibilities. Ethical considerations are part of daily practice. Acting with integrity is essential. It ensures that care remains patient-centered.

160. How do Clinical Pharmacists measure success in their role?

Success is measured through patient outcomes, safety improvements, and effective collaboration. Many contributions are not visible, but they are significant. Pharmacists often define success by the problems they prevent. Long-term impact matters more than immediate recognition. This perspective sustains commitment to the role.

161. How do Clinical Pharmacists build trust with physicians and nurses?

Trust is built through consistency, accuracy, and clear communication over time. When pharmacists provide reliable recommendations that improve outcomes, credibility grows naturally. Being responsive and respectful in interactions also strengthens relationships. Admitting uncertainty when appropriate reinforces honesty. Trust is earned through repeated, dependable performance.

162. How do Clinical Pharmacists handle being wrong?

They acknowledge it quickly, correct it, and learn from it. The focus is on patient safety and preventing recurrence, not protecting ego. Mistakes are reviewed constructively to improve systems and personal practice. Transparency builds trust within the team. Growth in pharmacy often comes from these moments.

163. What is the role of humility in pharmacy practice?

Humility keeps pharmacists open to learning and collaboration. It prevents overconfidence, which can lead to errors. Even experienced pharmacists recognize that medicine is constantly evolving. Asking questions and seeking input are signs of strength, not weakness. Humility supports safe, thoughtful care.

164. How do Clinical Pharmacists deal with difficult coworkers?

They maintain professionalism, focus on patient care, and communicate clearly. Personal differences are set aside to ensure safe and effective collaboration. When needed, concerns are addressed through appropriate channels. Strong communication skills help reduce tension. The priority remains the patient, not the conflict.

165. What is the importance of adaptability in pharmacy?

Adaptability allows pharmacists to respond effectively to changing conditions, such as new guidelines or unexpected patient needs. The healthcare environment is dynamic, and rigid thinking can limit effectiveness. Being flexible helps maintain performance under varying circumstances. Adaptability also supports long-term career growth. It is a key trait for success.

166. How do Clinical Pharmacists handle high expectations?

They rely on preparation, organization, and consistent performance to meet expectations. Understanding the scope of responsibility helps maintain focus. Over time, expectations become part of the standard rather than a source of pressure. Support from colleagues can also help manage demands. Meeting expectations requires both skill and discipline.

167. What is the role of resilience in pharmacy?

Resilience helps pharmacists recover from challenging situations and maintain performance over time. The profession involves stress, responsibility, and occasional setbacks. Developing resilience allows individuals to continue functioning effectively. It also supports long-term sustainability in the field. Resilience is built through experience and self-awareness.

168. How do Clinical Pharmacists stay motivated?

Motivation often comes from understanding the impact of their work on patient safety and outcomes. Even when recognition is limited, the knowledge of preventing harm provides purpose. Personal goals and professional growth also contribute to motivation. Supportive work environments can enhance engagement. Staying connected to purpose sustains motivation.

169. What is the role of curiosity in pharmacy practice?

Curiosity drives learning and improves clinical decision-making. Pharmacists who ask questions and seek deeper understanding are more effective. It helps identify potential issues that might otherwise be missed. Curiosity also supports adaptation to new information. It is a valuable trait for continuous improvement.

170. How do Clinical Pharmacists manage mental fatigue?

They use structured routines, brief mental breaks, and effective time management to reduce fatigue. Recognizing early signs of fatigue helps prevent errors. Support from colleagues can also provide relief during demanding periods. Maintaining balance outside of work is important. Managing fatigue is essential for safe practice.

171. What is the importance of consistency in pharmacy?

Consistency ensures that safety standards are maintained across all tasks. Reliable processes reduce variability and the risk of errors. Patients benefit from predictable, high-quality care. Consistency also builds trust within the healthcare team. It is a cornerstone of effective practice.

172. How do Clinical Pharmacists handle repetitive tasks without losing focus?

They rely on discipline and structured workflows to maintain attention. Even routine tasks are treated with importance because errors can occur at any level. Periodic mental resets help sustain focus. Experience also improves efficiency without reducing accuracy. Repetition becomes manageable with the right approach.

173. What is the role of self-awareness in pharmacy practice?

Self-awareness helps pharmacists recognize their strengths, limitations, and areas for growth. It allows them to seek support when needed and avoid overconfidence. Understanding personal tendencies improves decision-making. Self-awareness also supports emotional regulation. It is an important part of professional development.

174. How do Clinical Pharmacists balance confidence and caution?

They develop confidence through knowledge and experience while maintaining caution through consistent verification. Confidence allows for efficient decision-making, while caution ensures safety. The balance between the two is essential. Overconfidence can lead to errors, while excessive hesitation can slow care. Experience helps refine this balance.

175. What is the role of reflection in pharmacy practice?

Reflection allows pharmacists to review their decisions and identify areas for improvement. It supports continuous learning and growth. Reflecting on both successes and challenges provides valuable insights. This process strengthens clinical judgment over time. Reflection is a key component of professional development.

176. How do Clinical Pharmacists handle ambiguity in guidelines?

They interpret guidelines using clinical judgment and patient-specific factors. Not all situations are clearly defined, requiring flexibility in application. Collaboration with colleagues can help clarify decisions. Pharmacists must balance adherence to guidelines with individualized care. Managing ambiguity is part of advanced practice.

177. What is the impact of environment on job satisfaction?

The work environment significantly influences how the role feels on a daily basis. Supportive teams and adequate resources improve satisfaction. High-stress or understaffed environments can increase frustration. Alignment between personal preferences and the environment is critical. Job satisfaction often depends more on setting than role.

178. How do Clinical Pharmacists manage competing priorities?

They continuously reassess tasks based on urgency and importance. High-risk and time-sensitive issues take precedence. Effective prioritization requires both experience and situational awareness. Clear communication helps manage expectations. Managing priorities is a daily responsibility.

179. What is the importance of reliability in pharmacy practice?

Reliability ensures that others can depend on the pharmacist's work and recommendations. Consistent performance builds trust within the healthcare team. Unreliable practices increase risk and reduce effectiveness. Reliability supports both patient safety and professional credibility. It is a fundamental expectation.

180. How do Clinical Pharmacists handle long-term career growth?

They pursue additional training, certifications, or specialized roles based on their interests. Career growth often involves expanding responsibilities or transitioning to new settings. Continuous learning supports advancement. Networking and mentorship can also open opportunities. Growth is an ongoing process.

181. What is the role of accountability in pharmacy?

Accountability ensures that pharmacists take responsibility for their decisions and actions. It reinforces the importance of accuracy and ethical practice. Being accountable builds trust and credibility. It also supports a culture of safety. Accountability is central to professional responsibility.

182. How do Clinical Pharmacists manage expectations from leadership?

They align their work with organizational goals while maintaining focus on patient safety. Clear communication with leadership helps set realistic expectations. Understanding priorities allows for better performance. Support from leadership can enhance effectiveness. Managing expectations requires both clarity and adaptability.

183. What is the importance of efficiency in pharmacy practice?

Efficiency allows pharmacists to manage workload without

compromising accuracy. Streamlined processes improve productivity and reduce stress. However, efficiency must never come at the expense of safety. The goal is to work effectively, not just quickly. Balance is key.

184. How do Clinical Pharmacists stay engaged in their work?

Engagement comes from finding meaning in daily tasks and understanding their impact. Variety in responsibilities can also enhance interest. Opportunities for learning and growth contribute to engagement. Supportive environments encourage sustained involvement. Staying engaged helps prevent burnout.

185. What is the role of long-term perspective in pharmacy?

A long-term perspective helps pharmacists focus on sustainability rather than short-term performance. It allows for better career decisions and improved work-life balance. Understanding that growth takes time reduces pressure. This perspective supports resilience and satisfaction. It is important for lasting success.

186. How do Clinical Pharmacists maintain attention over long shifts?

They rely on structured workflows, habits, and periodic mental resets to sustain focus. Even brief pauses can help restore attention. Recognizing when concentration is slipping is critical to preventing errors. Experience helps build endurance over time. Maintaining focus is essential for patient safety.

187. What is the role of discipline in pharmacy practice?

Discipline ensures that processes are followed consistently, even under pressure. It reinforces accuracy and reduces the risk of shortcuts. Pharmacists depend on disciplined habits to maintain performance. This consistency supports patient safety and reliability. Discipline is a defining characteristic of effective practice.

188. How do Clinical Pharmacists respond to unexpected challenges?

They assess the situation quickly, gather available information, and apply clinical judgment. Flexibility and calm decision-making are key. Collaboration with the care team often helps resolve complex issues. Experience improves response time and confidence. Unexpected challenges are a regular part of the role.

189. What is the importance of clarity in communication?

Clarity ensures that recommendations are understood and followed correctly. Miscommunication can lead to errors or delays in care. Pharmacists must express complex ideas in simple, direct terms. Clear communication builds trust and efficiency. It is essential in all interactions.

190. How do Clinical Pharmacists build confidence in their role?

Confidence develops through experience, repetition, and successful outcomes. Learning from both successes and challenges strengthens self-assurance. Support from colleagues also contributes to confidence. Over time, familiarity with clinical situations reduces hesitation. Confidence must always be balanced with caution.

191. What is the role of patience in pharmacy practice?

Patience allows pharmacists to work through complex problems without rushing. It is especially important when dealing with patients or challenging situations. Taking the time to understand details improves outcomes. Patience also supports effective communication. It is a key trait for long-term success.

192. How do Clinical Pharmacists maintain ethical standards?

They follow professional guidelines, prioritize patient safety, and act with integrity. Ethical decision-making is part of daily practice. Pharmacists must balance multiple responsibilities while maintaining standards. Transparency and accountability support ethical behavior. Ethics guide actions in complex situations.

193. What is the importance of precision in pharmacy?

Precision ensures that medications are used safely and effectively. Small errors can have significant consequences. Pharmacists develop habits that reinforce accuracy in all tasks. This attention to detail is critical for patient safety. Precision defines the profession.

194. How do Clinical Pharmacists stay calm under pressure?

They rely on training, preparation, and controlled responses to manage stress. Staying calm allows for clearer thinking and better decisions. Experience helps reduce emotional reactions to pressure. Structured processes provide stability in high-stress situations. Calmness is essential for effective performance.

195. What is the role of continuous improvement in pharmacy?

Continuous improvement involves refining processes, learning from experiences, and adapting to new information. Pharmacists constantly evaluate their performance. This mindset supports better outcomes over time. Improvement is not occasional—it is ongoing. It is a key part of professional growth.

196. How do Clinical Pharmacists handle responsibility for patient outcomes?

They accept responsibility as part of the role while focusing on doing their best with available information. Not all outcomes are within their control, but their contribution matters. This responsibility can be heavy, especially early in a career. Over time, it becomes integrated into daily practice. Managing this responsibility is essential for sustainability.

197. What is the importance of trust in pharmacy practice?

Trust allows the healthcare team to rely on the pharmacist's expertise. It also supports patient confidence in medication use. Building trust requires consistency and professionalism. Without trust, collaboration becomes difficult. It is a fundamental element of effective care.

198. How do Clinical Pharmacists maintain work-life balance?

They set boundaries, manage time effectively, and prioritize activities outside of work. Balance varies depending on the role and setting. Supportive environments make balance easier to achieve. Recognizing limits helps prevent burnout. Maintaining balance is important for long-term success.

199. What is the role of purpose in pharmacy practice?

Purpose provides motivation and direction in daily work. Understanding the impact of their role helps pharmacists stay engaged. Purpose connects routine tasks to meaningful outcomes. It reinforces commitment during challenging times. A strong sense of purpose supports resilience.

200. How do Clinical Pharmacists define long-term success?

Long-term success is defined by sustained performance, growth, and positive patient outcomes. It involves developing expertise and maintaining alignment with the role. Recognition may vary, but impact remains consistent. Success is not a single achievement—it is ongoing. It reflects both professional and personal fulfillment.

201. What is the most important quality for a Clinical Pharmacist to have?

Attention to detail combined with accountability is essential. These qualities ensure that decisions are both accurate and responsible. Without them, patient safety is at risk. While many skills are important, these form the foundation. They support all other aspects of the role.

202. If you could summarize the role of a Clinical Pharmacist in one sentence, what would it be?

A Clinical Pharmacist is the final safeguard in medication use, combining knowledge, precision, and judgment to ensure that every therapy is as safe and effective as possible.

3

THE TOLL BOOTH™

The Emotional, Cognitive, and Lifestyle Cost of Becoming a Clinical Pharmacist

Every healthcare career has a cost.

Not just in time.

Not just in money.

But in how the work shapes you—mentally, emotionally, and over time.

That cost is what we call **The Toll Booth™**.

And for Clinical Pharmacists, the toll is rarely obvious from the outside.

Because on paper, this role looks stable, respected, and intellectually rewarding. It is often positioned as a "safer" or more sustainable alternative to other clinical paths—less physically demanding than nursing, more structured than physician training, and deeply rooted in science and precision.

All of that is true.

But it is not the whole truth.

The real toll of this role lives in what you carry quietly.

. . .

The Weight of Being the Final Check

In many healthcare environments, the Clinical Pharmacist is the last line of defense between a medication order and a patient.

That sounds straightforward.

Until you realize what it actually means.

You are responsible for catching:

- Incorrect dosages
- Dangerous drug interactions
- Allergies that were missed
- Contraindications that could cause harm
- Subtle clinical details others may have overlooked

Most of the time, nothing happens.

Because you caught it.

And when nothing happens, no one notices.

But when something does happen—even rarely—the consequences can be severe.

This creates a unique kind of pressure:

You are expected to be perfect in a system that is not.

Over time, that responsibility becomes heavy—not because of what goes wrong, but because of what *could have* gone wrong.

The Cognitive Load of Constant Precision

Clinical Pharmacists operate in an environment where accuracy is not optional.

Every decision requires:

- Focus
- Attention to detail
- Clinical judgment
- Rapid verification

And unlike roles that allow for natural variation in pace, pharmacy work often demands **sustained precision over long periods of time.**

There is no "coasting."

There is no autopilot.

Even repetitive tasks carry risk.

Verifying the same type of order hundreds of times does not make it less important—it makes it easier to miss something.

That mental strain adds up.

Not in dramatic spikes—but in quiet, cumulative fatigue.

At the end of a shift, many Clinical Pharmacists don't feel physically exhausted.

They feel mentally drained in a way that is harder to explain—and harder to recover from.

The Invisible Nature of the Work

One of the most overlooked aspects of this career is how often the impact is unseen.

You may prevent harm multiple times in a single shift.

You may improve therapy, optimize dosing, and contribute meaningfully to patient outcomes.

And yet, patients often don't know your name.

Even within care teams, your role can be misunderstood or under-recognized depending on the setting.

In some environments, Clinical Pharmacists are fully integrated into rounds and decision-making.

In others, they operate more in the background—consulted when needed, but not always fully included.

This creates a tension between **high responsibility and low visibility.**

For some people, that's fine.

For others, it becomes a source of frustration over time.

Especially if part of your identity is tied to connection, recognition, or direct patient interaction.

Hierarchy and Interpersonal Friction

Healthcare is a team environment.

But it is not always an equal one.

Clinical Pharmacists frequently collaborate with physicians, nurses, and other providers—and in many cases, they must challenge or question orders to ensure safety.

That requires confidence, communication skills, and emotional intelligence.

Because not every interaction is easy.

There will be moments where:

- Your recommendations are questioned
- Your input is dismissed
- You have to advocate for a safer option despite resistance

These are not daily occurrences in every setting—but they are part of the reality.

And they require a specific kind of professional resilience:

The ability to speak up without escalating conflict.

The ability to stay grounded even when others are not.

The ability to prioritize patient safety over personal comfort.

Over time, that dynamic can be either energizing or exhausting—depending on your personality and the culture you work in.

Retail vs. Clinical: Two Different Tolls

Not all pharmacy roles carry the same burden.

Retail pharmacy often involves:

- High prescription volume
- Time pressure
- Customer-facing stress
- Insurance and billing frustrations
- Limited staffing

The toll here is often **speed + volume + interruption.**

Clinical pharmacy, especially in hospital or specialty settings, shifts the toll toward:

- Cognitive intensity
- Clinical responsibility
- Interdisciplinary dynamics
- Decision-making under uncertainty

The stress is different.

Less transactional.

More analytical.

But no less real.

Understanding which type of toll aligns—or conflicts—with your personality is critical.

Ethical Tension and System Constraints

Clinical Pharmacists often sit at the intersection of clinical care and system limitations.

You may know the optimal therapy for a patient.

But that therapy may not be:

- Covered by insurance
- Available in your formulary
- Affordable for the patient

This creates ethical friction.

You are trained to optimize care.

But you are also operating within constraints that don't always allow for ideal decisions.

Over time, that gap between *what should be done* and *what can be done* can wear on people—especially those who are highly patient-centered.

The Accumulation Effect

None of these pressures, on their own, define the career.

In fact, many Clinical Pharmacists find their work deeply meaningful, intellectually engaging, and professionally fulfilling.

But The Toll Booth™ is not about isolated moments.

It's about accumulation.

- The mental fatigue from sustained precision
- The quiet pressure of being the safety net
- The frustration of limited visibility
- The emotional effort of navigating hierarchy

• The ethical tension of constrained systems

Over months and years, these factors either align with who you are...

Or they don't.

Alignment Matters More Than Capability

You can be highly intelligent, detail-oriented, and academically successful—and still find this role draining if it does not align with your identity.

This is where Mason's Alignment Theory (MAT) becomes essential.

Using **PACES™** (Personality, Aptitude, Constraints, Experience, Situation) and **CARESET™** (Culture, Autonomy, Resources, Expectations, Environment, Team), the question is not:

"Can you do this job?"

It is:

"Does this job fit how you are wired—and what you need to sustain it over time?"

Because the Clinical Pharmacist role rewards:

• Precision
• Consistency
• Analytical thinking
• Comfort with indirect impact
• Willingness to operate in structured systems

If that aligns with you, the toll is manageable—and often worth it.

If it doesn't, the same responsibilities that make the role important can become the very things that make it difficult to sustain.

The Honest Takeaway

Becoming a Clinical Pharmacist is not just a professional decision.

It is a long-term commitment to a specific type of work, pressure, and responsibility.

There is pride in this role.

There is purpose in this role.

But there is also a cost.

And the more clearly you understand that cost now...

The better equipped you will be to decide whether it is the right path for you.

4

THE COGNITIVE LOAD OF BEING A CLINICAL PHARMACIST

5

MONEY MAP™

What It Looks Like in Real Life (Expanded Scenarios)

The numbers tell part of the story.

But numbers alone don't show what the experience feels like over time.

To understand the financial reality of becoming a Clinical Pharmacist, it helps to look at how different paths actually unfold—month by month, year by year.

These are not perfect projections.

They are realistic scenarios based on common paths pharmacists take.

Scenario 1 — The Immediate Earner (Retail Path)

You graduate, pass your boards, and step directly into a full-time retail pharmacist role.

Your starting salary feels strong—often in the range of $115,000 to $130,000.

On paper, it looks like you've "made it."

But your financial life quickly becomes more complex than the number suggests.

You begin managing:

• Student loan payments that may exceed $1,500–$2,000 per month

• A demanding schedule that limits flexibility

• A pace of work that can feel constant and difficult to step away from

In the first two years, income is high—but so is the pressure.

You are earning, but you are also adjusting.

By years 3–5, you may begin to stabilize financially, especially if you are aggressive with debt repayment.

But this is also when a different question begins to surface:

Is this pace something I want to sustain long-term?

For some pharmacists, the answer is yes.

For others, this becomes the moment where financial success and lifestyle begin to feel misaligned.

Scenario 2 — **The Delayed Builder (Clinical Residency Path)**

You choose a different route.

Instead of entering the workforce immediately at full salary, you pursue residency training.

Your income during this time is significantly lower—often between $50,000 and $60,000.

At the same time, your debt does not pause.

Interest continues to accumulate.

Financially, this can feel like you are moving backward while others are moving forward.

But what you are building is not immediate income—it is positioning.

After completing residency, you transition into a clinical role.

Your salary may now fall in the range of $110,000 to $135,000.

While you may still be behind the retail path in total earnings, something else has changed:

Your options have expanded.

You may now have access to:

• Specialized clinical roles
• Academic positions
• Leadership pathways

Over time, the gap between early earnings begins to matter less.

The question becomes:

Did this path create a career that feels more aligned—and therefore more sustainable?

Scenario 3 — The Strategic Pivot (Industry Transition)

You begin your career in a traditional setting—retail or clinical—and then make a strategic shift.

This transition often does not happen immediately.

It requires:

• Experience
• Networking
• Positioning yourself for a different type of role

When you enter the pharmaceutical industry, your income may increase significantly.

Salaries in this space often range from $130,000 to $180,000 or more, depending on the role.

But the nature of the work changes.

You move from:

• Individual patient care

to

• Broader impact across populations

The stress is different.

Instead of workflow pressure, you may experience:

• Performance expectations
• Travel demands
• Strategic responsibilities

Financially, this path can be highly rewarding.

But the alignment question shifts:

Do you want your impact to be direct—or distributed?

. . .

What These Paths Have in Common

Despite their differences, these scenarios share a few important realities:

1 Debt is a constant early factor

No matter the path, student loans influence your first several years.

2 Income alone does not determine satisfaction

Higher pay does not automatically mean better alignment.

3 Early decisions shape long-term flexibility

Residency, specialization, and experience all influence future options.

4 Lifestyle matters as much as salary

The day-to-day experience of your work shapes how that income feels.

The Financial Reality Most People Miss

Many people enter pharmacy focusing on one number:

👉 Starting salary

But the real financial experience is shaped by:

- Time (how long it takes to reach stability)
- Energy (how demanding the work feels)
- Flexibility (how easily you can adjust your path)
- Sustainability (whether you can maintain it long-term)

Two pharmacists can earn the same income...

And have completely different financial experiences based on those factors.

Bringing It Back to Alignment

This is where Money Map™ connects directly to Mason's Alignment Theory (MAT).

Using:

- **PACES™**
- **CARESET™**

You are not just asking:

👉 "Does this career pay well?"

You are asking:

👉 **"Does this financial path fit the life I want to live?"**

Because the goal is not just to earn.

It is to build something you can sustain—financially, emotionally, and professionally.

6

TERMS OF CARE™

Terms of Care™

Compensation in healthcare is rarely as simple as a base salary, and Clinical Pharmacy is no exception. What is offered on paper is only one part of the total picture. Understanding the full scope of compensation, benefits, expectations, and tradeoffs is essential before accepting any role. Too many professionals focus only on the salary number and overlook the broader structure that ultimately defines their experience.

Base salary for Clinical Pharmacists can vary depending on setting, geography, and level of specialization. Hospital-based roles, ambulatory care positions, and specialty areas such as oncology or critical care may offer different compensation ranges. Experience, residency training, and board certification can also influence earning potential. While salary is important, it should always be evaluated in context with the rest of the offer.

Benefits are a significant component of total compensation, often representing a substantial portion of the overall package. Health insurance, retirement contributions, paid time off, and continuing education support all contribute to the real value of a position. In many healthcare systems, benefits can represent a meaningful percentage of what the employer is investing in you. Evaluating these details carefully can prevent surprises after you begin the role.

Work schedule and expectations are another critical part of the Terms of Care™. Some positions require rotating shifts, weekends, or holidays, while others offer more predictable hours. Staffing models, workload expectations, and coverage requirements can significantly affect your day-to-day experience. A higher salary may not feel worth it if the schedule leads to burnout or limits your ability to maintain a sustainable routine.

Professional development support should also be considered. Opportunities for continuing education, certifications, conference attendance, and career advancement can shape your long-term trajectory. Some organizations invest heavily in the growth of their pharmacists, while others provide minimal support. Understanding what is available—and what is expected of you in return—is essential.

Another important factor is the structure of the team and the resources available to you. Adequate staffing, access to technology, and supportive leadership all influence your ability to perform effectively. Even a well-paying role can become challenging if resources are limited or expectations are unrealistic. The environment in which you work will ultimately determine how sustainable the position feels.

Loan repayment and financial obligations are also part of the equation. Many pharmacists graduate with significant educational debt, and repayment structures can influence career decisions. Some employers offer loan assistance programs or incentives, while others do not. Evaluating how your compensation aligns with your financial responsibilities is a critical step in making an informed decision.

It is also important to understand what success looks like in the role. Performance expectations, evaluation criteria, and opportunities for advancement should be clearly defined. Knowing how you will be assessed helps you align your efforts with the goals of the organization. It also provides clarity on how you can grow within the position over time.

Negotiation is often underutilized in healthcare roles, but it is an important part of the process. While not every element of an offer is flexible, there may be opportunities to adjust aspects such as salary, schedule, or professional development support. Approaching negotiation with professionalism and preparation can lead to a more balanced and sustainable agreement.

Ultimately, the Terms of Care™ represent more than just compensation—they define the structure of your professional life. A role that looks attractive on the surface may not align with your long-term goals if the underlying terms are not supportive. Taking the time to evaluate each component carefully allows you to make decisions that are not only financially sound, but also aligned with your overall well-being.

Choosing a Clinical Pharmacist role is not just about accepting a job. It is about entering into an agreement that will shape your daily experience, your growth, and your sustainability in the profession. Understanding the full Terms of Care™ ensures that you are making that decision with clarity and confidence.

7

FIT ANALYZER™

SCRUBfit™ Role Fit Index (RFI): Clinical Pharmacist

Up to this point, you've explored what the Clinical Pharmacist role looks like, what it costs emotionally and financially, and how it plays out across different settings.

Now comes the most important question:

Does this role actually fit you?

Not on paper.

Not based on what you're capable of.

But based on how you are wired—and what you need to sustain a career over time.

This is where the **SCRUBfit™ Role Fit Index (RFI)** comes in.

This is not a test.

There are no right or wrong answers.

It is a mirror.

How to Use This Tool

Below are 15 statements based on real-world Clinical Pharmacist responsibilities, environments, and pressures.

For each statement, rate yourself on a scale from **1 to 10:**

- **1 = Strongly Disagree**
- **10 = Strongly Agree**

Answer honestly—not aspirationally.

This works best when you reflect who you are *right now*, not who you think you should be.

SCRUBFIT™ ROLE Fit Index Statements — Clinical Pharmacist

1 I am comfortable being responsible for patient outcomes even when I am not the one directly prescribing medications.

2 I can maintain a high level of focus and accuracy during repetitive, detail-oriented tasks.

3 I enjoy analyzing complex information and making precise, evidence-based recommendations.

4 I am comfortable working in structured systems with protocols, guidelines, and defined workflows.

5 I can handle situations where my contributions may not be highly visible, even when they are impactful.

6 I am willing to speak up and advocate for patient safety, even if it means questioning another provider's decision.

7 I can manage mental fatigue that comes from sustained concentration over long periods of time.

8 I am comfortable with indirect patient impact rather than constant face-to-face interaction.

9 I value accuracy and safety more than speed or high variability in my work environment.

10 I can handle occasional interpersonal friction in a professional setting without becoming disengaged.

11 I am willing to continue learning and adapting as medications, technologies, and guidelines evolve.

12 I can tolerate working within system constraints, even when I know the ideal solution may not be possible.

13 I am comfortable with a career path that may require additional training (such as residency) to access certain roles.

14 I prefer environments where attention to detail is critical and

mistakes can have serious consequences.

15 I can see myself sustaining this type of work—not just for a few years, but over the long term.

Scoring Your Results

Add up your total score.

- **Maximum Score:** 150
- **Minimum Score:** 15

Understanding Your Score

120–150: High Alignment

Your responses suggest a strong alignment with the Clinical Pharmacist role.

You likely:

- Value precision and structured environments
- Are comfortable with responsibility and indirect impact
- Can sustain the cognitive demands of the role

This doesn't guarantee the path will be easy—but it does suggest the core nature of the work fits how you are wired.

90–119: Partial Alignment

There are elements of this role that may fit you well—and others that may not.

This is where setting becomes critical.

For example:

- You may prefer more patient-facing roles (ambulatory care) over more operational ones
- You may thrive in collaborative teams but struggle in more hierarchical environments

This range requires deeper reflection and intentional career shaping.

. . .

Below 90: Potential Misalignment

Your responses suggest that key aspects of the Clinical Pharmacist role may not align with your natural preferences or long-term needs.

This does not mean you *can't* do the job.

It means the day-to-day realities may feel draining over time.

In many cases, people in this range succeed academically—but struggle with long-term sustainability and satisfaction.

The Reflection That Matters Most

Numbers help.

But the real value comes from this question:

Which statements gave you pause—and why?

Those moments of hesitation are often more important than your total score.

They point to:

- Potential friction points
- Areas of misalignment
- Aspects of the role that may require more energy to sustain

Pay attention to them.

Alignment Over Capability

This tool is grounded in Mason's Alignment Theory (MAT), using:

- **PACES™** (Personality, Aptitude, Constraints, Experience, Situation)
- **CARESET™** (Culture, Autonomy, Resources, Expectations, Environment, Team)

The goal is not to determine whether you *can* become a Clinical Pharmacist.

It is to explore whether you can become one **and still feel like yourself over time.**

Because capability can get you into a role.

Only alignment keeps you there.

. . .

The Honest Takeaway

The Clinical Pharmacist role is:

- Intellectually demanding
- Detail-driven
- High in responsibility
- Often low in visibility

For the right person, that combination is deeply satisfying.

For the wrong fit, it can feel quietly exhausting.

The difference is not talent.

It is alignment.

And the more clearly you see that now...

The more confident—and intentional—your next decision will be.

8

PIVOT PLAYBOOK™

How Clinical Pharmacists Adapt, Transition, and Redesign Their Careers Over Time

Very few healthcare careers are linear.

And pharmacy is no exception.

While the path to becoming a Clinical Pharmacist can feel structured—undergraduate coursework, PharmD, residency, and then practice—the reality is that many pharmacists adjust, pivot, or completely redesign their careers over time.

That is not failure.

That is adaptation.

This section is about understanding your options—before you need them.

Because the most confident career decisions are made by people who know:

If this path changes... I still have a path.

Why Pharmacists Pivot

Clinical Pharmacists choose to pivot for a variety of reasons:

- Burnout from sustained cognitive load or workflow pressure

- Desire for more patient interaction—or less
- Frustration with system constraints or limited autonomy
- Interest in business, industry, or non-clinical roles
- Lifestyle shifts (family, schedule, location flexibility)

Sometimes the pivot is proactive.

Sometimes it is reactive.

Either way, it is common.

And often, it is necessary for long-term alignment.

Pivot Path #1 — Retail to Clinical

This is one of the most common transitions in pharmacy.

Many pharmacists begin in retail settings and later seek more clinically integrated roles.

Why people make this move:

- High prescription volume and workflow pressure
- Customer-facing stress and interruptions
- Desire for deeper clinical involvement

What it often requires:

- Additional experience or certifications
- In some cases, residency (though not always)
- Networking and persistence

The tradeoff:

- Potential decrease in starting salary
- Increase in clinical engagement and team-based care

For many, this pivot improves alignment—even if it requires short-term sacrifice.

Pivot Path #2 — Clinical to Specialized Practice

After entering clinical roles, some pharmacists choose to specialize.

Common areas include:

- Oncology
- Infectious disease

- Cardiology
- Critical care
- Ambulatory care

Why this path appeals:

- Deeper expertise
- Increased clinical impact
- Greater integration with medical teams

What it often requires:

- PGY2 residency or equivalent experience
- Board certification (e.g., BCPS, BCOP)

The tradeoff:

- Additional training time
- Higher expectations and responsibility

For those who enjoy complexity and depth, this can be a highly rewarding path.

PIVOT PATH #3 — Clinical to Pharmaceutical Industry

Some Clinical Pharmacists transition into roles within the pharmaceutical industry.

Common positions include:

- Medical Science Liaison (MSL)
- Medical Affairs
- Clinical Research
- Drug Safety / Pharmacovigilance

Why this path appeals:

- Higher earning potential
- Reduced clinical workflow pressure
- Strategic, education-focused work

What it requires:

- Strong communication and presentation skills
- Willingness to travel (for some roles)
- A shift from direct patient care to broader impact

The tradeoff:

- Less direct patient interaction

• Different performance expectations and metrics

This path often attracts those who enjoy science, communication, and big-picture impact.

Pivot Path #4 — Clinical to Non-Clinical Roles

Pharmacy training opens doors beyond traditional patient care.

Some pharmacists transition into:

• Informatics
• Medication safety and quality improvement
• Healthcare consulting
• Policy and regulatory roles
• Education and academia

Why this path appeals:

• New intellectual challenges
• Broader system-level impact
• Alternative work environments

The tradeoff:

• May require additional training or experience
• Less traditional "clinical" identity

For some, this pivot provides a better long-term fit—especially if direct clinical work becomes draining.

Pivot Path #5 — Redesigning Within the Role

Not every pivot requires leaving clinical practice.

Sometimes the shift happens within the role itself.

Examples include:

• Moving from inpatient to ambulatory care
• Transitioning from high-intensity settings (ICU) to more structured environments
• Adjusting schedules (full-time to part-time)
• Seeking organizations with better culture or support

This type of pivot is often overlooked.

But it can be one of the most effective ways to restore alignment without starting over.

The Cost of Waiting Too Long

One of the biggest risks in any career is staying in a misaligned role for too long.

Over time, this can lead to:

- Burnout
- Reduced performance or engagement
- Loss of confidence
- Financial and emotional strain

The longer you wait, the harder it can feel to change.

Not because the options disappear.

But because the energy required to pursue them increases.

What Makes a Pivot Successful

Successful pivots are rarely random.

They are intentional.

They involve:

- Honest self-assessment
- Willingness to learn or retrain
- Strategic networking
- Financial planning

And most importantly:

They are guided by alignment—not just escape.

Because leaving one misaligned role for another does not solve the problem.

It just moves it.

Using Alignment as Your Compass

This is where Mason's Alignment Theory (MAT) becomes practical.

Using:

• **PACES™** (Personality, Aptitude, Constraints, Experience, Situation)

• **CARESET™** (Culture, Autonomy, Resources, Expectations, Environment, Team)

You can evaluate not just whether a new path is possible—

But whether it is a better fit.

Each pivot should move you closer to:

- Work that fits how you think
- Environments that support how you operate
- Responsibilities that feel sustainable over time

The Honest Takeaway

The Clinical Pharmacist path is not a single road.

It is a network of pathways—some expected, some less obvious.

You may stay in one lane for your entire career.

Or you may shift directions more than once.

Both are valid.

What matters is not whether you pivot.

It is whether your path—wherever it leads—continues to align with who you are.

Because the goal is not just to build a career.

It is to build one you can live with.

9

TECHNOLOGY AND INNOVATION™

Navigating the Digital Transformation of Clinical Pharmacy

Clinical pharmacy is not what it was even ten years ago.

And it will not look the same ten years from now.

Technology is rapidly reshaping how medications are prescribed, verified, dispensed, monitored, and optimized. For Clinical Pharmacists, this shift is not optional—it is part of the role.

Understanding how technology fits into your daily work is no longer a bonus skill.

It is a core competency.

The Modern Clinical Environment

Today's Clinical Pharmacists operate within complex digital ecosystems that include:

- Electronic Health Records (EHRs)
- Clinical decision support tools
- Automated dispensing systems
- Medication safety alerts

- Telehealth and remote care platforms

These systems are designed to improve safety, efficiency, and coordination.

But they also introduce new challenges—especially around workflow, alert fatigue, and information overload.

Electronic Health Records (EHRs)

Most Clinical Pharmacists work within EHR systems such as Epic, Cerner, or Athenahealth.

These platforms are central to:

- Reviewing medication orders
- Accessing patient histories
- Monitoring lab results
- Documenting interventions

Efficiency in these systems matters.

Small improvements in navigation, documentation, and workflow can significantly reduce cognitive load over the course of a shift.

At the same time, EHRs can contribute to:

- Screen fatigue
- Documentation burden
- Fragmented attention

Learning to use these tools effectively—and setting boundaries around their use—is part of long-term sustainability.

Clinical Decision Support Systems

Clinical decision support tools are built into many pharmacy workflows.

These systems provide:

- Drug interaction alerts
- Dosing recommendations
- Allergy checks
- Clinical guidelines

They are designed to reduce error.

But they are not perfect.

One of the most common challenges is **alert fatigue**—the experience of being presented with so many warnings that it becomes difficult to distinguish critical issues from routine notifications.

Clinical Pharmacists must learn to:

- Interpret alerts critically
- Avoid over-reliance on automation
- Maintain independent clinical judgment

Technology supports decision-making.

It does not replace it.

AUTOMATION AND DISPENSING Technology

In many settings, medication distribution is supported by automated systems such as:

- Automated dispensing cabinets (ADCs)
- Robotic packaging systems
- Centralized medication distribution technologies

These systems improve:

- Efficiency
- Inventory control
- Medication tracking

They also shift the role of the pharmacist.

Less time is spent on manual dispensing.

More time is spent on:

- Verification
- Clinical oversight
- Problem-solving

This transition reinforces the identity of the Clinical Pharmacist as a **clinical decision-maker**, not just a dispenser.

TELEPHARMACY AND REMOTE Care

Telepharmacy is expanding access to pharmacy services—especially in rural and underserved areas.

Through remote systems, Clinical Pharmacists can:

- Verify medication orders
- Consult with providers
- Support patient care from a distance

This model offers:

- Increased flexibility
- Broader reach
- New employment structures

But it also introduces:

- Reduced in-person interaction
- Dependence on technology infrastructure
- Potential communication challenges

For some pharmacists, this is an exciting shift.

For others, it may feel disconnected from traditional clinical environments.

Artificial Intelligence and Predictive Tools

Artificial intelligence (AI) is beginning to influence clinical pharmacy in meaningful ways.

Emerging tools can:

- Analyze large datasets for medication trends
- Identify potential adverse events earlier
- Support clinical decision-making
- Optimize medication therapy at scale

These technologies are still evolving.

And they raise important questions:

- How much should we rely on automated recommendations?
- Where does human judgment remain essential?
- How do we ensure safety in rapidly changing systems?

For Clinical Pharmacists, the future will likely involve working *with* AI—not being replaced by it.

Specialty Pharmacy and Complex Therapies

Advances in medication development—especially in biologics and specialty drugs—are transforming pharmacy practice.

Clinical Pharmacists are increasingly involved in:

- Managing high-cost therapies
- Coordinating prior authorizations
- Monitoring complex treatment regimens
- Educating patients and providers

These medications often require:

- Detailed tracking
- Ongoing monitoring
- Coordination across multiple systems

Technology supports this process—but also adds layers of complexity.

The Digital Workload

While technology improves many aspects of care, it also contributes to a different kind of workload:

- Multiple systems running simultaneously
- Constant notifications and alerts
- Rapid switching between tasks
- Increased documentation requirements

This creates a form of **digital fatigue** that is less visible than physical exhaustion—but just as real.

Learning to manage this environment is part of the job.

And it requires:

- Focus
- Workflow awareness
- Intentional use of technology

Staying **Current in a Moving Field**

Technology in healthcare evolves quickly.

New systems, updates, and tools are introduced regularly.

For Clinical Pharmacists, this means:

- Ongoing learning is required
- Adaptability is essential
- Comfort with change becomes an advantage

Those who resist change may struggle.

Those who engage with it—thoughtfully and critically—often find new opportunities.

ALIGNMENT IN A DIGITAL World

Not everyone enjoys technology-driven environments.

Some people thrive in:

- Structured, data-rich systems
- Analytical workflows
- Digitally integrated care models

Others prefer:

- Face-to-face interaction
- Less screen time
- More tangible, hands-on work

This is where alignment matters.

Using Mason's Alignment Theory (MAT), and applying **PACES™** and **CARESET™**, the question becomes:

Does this type of digital environment support how you think and work?

Because technology is not going away.

If anything, it will become more central to the role.

THE HONEST TAKEAWAY

Technology is transforming clinical pharmacy in powerful ways.

It is improving safety.

Expanding access.

Enhancing decision-making.

But it is also:

- Increasing cognitive load
- Changing how pharmacists interact with patients and teams

- Introducing new types of stress and fatigue

For the right person, this environment is engaging and intellectually rewarding.

For others, it may feel overwhelming or disconnected.

Understanding how you respond to technology—not just your ability to use it—is an important part of choosing this path.

Because the future of clinical pharmacy is not just clinical.

It is digital.

10

CAREERNAV™

How Clinical Pharmacists Actually Get Hired

Getting hired as a Clinical Pharmacist is not just about having the right degree or passing the required exams. It is about positioning yourself correctly in a highly competitive and often opaque hiring landscape. Many qualified candidates struggle not because they lack ability, but because they do not fully understand how hiring decisions are made within healthcare systems. Knowing how to navigate this process can significantly increase your chances of securing the right role.

Most Clinical Pharmacist roles are filled through a combination of formal applications and informal networks. Hospital and health-system career portals are the most visible entry point, but they are not always the most effective on their own. Many positions are influenced by internal referrals, prior rotations, or professional connections. This means that simply submitting applications online, while necessary, is rarely sufficient as a standalone strategy.

Your clinical rotations, residency experiences, and professional relationships play a major role in your candidacy. Preceptors, colleagues, and supervisors often serve as informal references long before an official reference check occurs. The impressions you leave during training can directly influence whether you are considered for future opportunities. This is why consistency, professionalism, and engagement during these experiences are critical.

Professional associations and organizations are another valuable resource. Groups related to pharmacy practice areas, such as hospital pharmacy or specialty disciplines, often provide networking opportunities, job boards, and industry insights. Engaging with these communities allows you to stay informed about trends and connect with professionals who may have knowledge of open positions before they are widely advertised.

Online job platforms such as LinkedIn and Indeed are commonly used in healthcare recruiting. These platforms allow you to search for roles, connect with recruiters, and present your professional profile. However, they should be viewed as tools rather than complete solutions. The most effective candidates use these platforms in combination with direct outreach and networking efforts.

Working with recruiters can also be part of the process, particularly for specialized or hard-to-fill roles. Recruiters may have access to positions that are not publicly posted and can help guide you through the hiring process. However, it is important to approach these relationships with clarity and professionalism. Not all recruiters operate the same way, and understanding their role in the process helps you set appropriate expectations.

Your resume plays a critical role in how you are initially evaluated. Healthcare systems often use applicant tracking systems (ATS) to screen candidates before a human review occurs. This means your resume must be structured in a way that is both clear and optimized for these systems. Including relevant keywords, highlighting clinical experience, and demonstrating measurable impact can improve your chances of moving forward.

Beyond the resume, your ability to communicate effectively with hiring managers is essential. Reaching out with thoughtful, concise messages that demonstrate interest and understanding of the role can set you apart. This is especially true when contacting pharmacy directors or clinical leaders directly. A well-crafted message can open doors that a standard application cannot.

Understanding the timeline of the hiring process is also important. Healthcare hiring can be slower than other industries due to approval processes, budgeting considerations, and internal coordination. Patience and persistence are required. Following up appropriately without becoming overly aggressive shows professionalism and continued interest.

It is also important to recognize that rejection is part of the process. Not every role will be the right fit, and not every application will lead to an offer. The goal is not to secure every opportunity, but to secure the right one. Learning from each experience and refining your approach will improve your results over time.

Ultimately, CareerNav™ is about more than finding a job. It is about understanding how the system works and positioning yourself within it effectively. When you combine strong clinical preparation with strategic navigation of the hiring process, you increase your chances of finding a role that aligns with both your skills and your long-term goals.

11

PROFESSIONAL DEVELOPMENT ROADMAP™

Planning Your Clinical Pharmacist Career Trajectory

Becoming a Clinical Pharmacist is not a single decision.

It is a series of decisions made over time.

What you do in your first year matters.

What you build by year five matters more.

And what you sustain over ten years determines the kind of career—and life—you ultimately create.

This is where the **Professional Development Roadmap™** comes in.

Not as a rigid plan.

But as a way to think strategically about your growth—so your career evolves with intention, not by default.

The First Year — Transitioning From Student to Practitioner

The first year of practice is one of the most important—and most underestimated—phases of your career.

Whether you enter through residency or directly into a role, this period is about:

- Building confidence in real-world decision-making

- Translating knowledge into practice
- Learning workflow, systems, and expectations
- Developing professional relationships

This is also where many new Clinical Pharmacists experience their first true exposure to the pace and pressure of the role.

Mistakes feel heavier.

Uncertainty feels more frequent.

Responsibility feels real.

The goal during this phase is not perfection.

It is **adaptation.**

Years Two to Five — **Building Competence and Identity**

Once the initial transition period passes, the focus shifts toward establishing yourself.

This is where you begin to answer:

- What type of Clinical Pharmacist do I want to be?
- Which settings or specialties fit me best?
- What aspects of the work energize me—and which drain me?

During this phase, many pharmacists pursue:

- Board certification (such as BCPS or specialty certifications)
- Deeper involvement in clinical teams
- Expanded responsibilities or leadership within their department

This is also a critical window for alignment.

If the role or environment does not fit, this is often when that realization becomes clear.

And it is the right time to adjust—not after years of misalignment.

Years Five to Ten — **Specialization and Leadership**

By this stage, your career begins to take shape.

You may choose to:

• Deepen your expertise in a specialty area (oncology, infectious disease, critical care)

• Move into supervisory or leadership roles

• Transition into education, research, or program development

You are no longer just learning the role.

You are shaping it.

This phase often brings:

• Greater autonomy

• Increased expectations

• Broader influence within your organization

It also brings a new question:

Do you want to go deeper—or broader?

Beyond Ten Years — **Sustainability and Redesign**

Long-term careers in clinical pharmacy require sustainability.

This is where many professionals begin to reassess:

• Is my current role still aligned with who I am?

• Do I want to continue at this pace or level of intensity?

• Are there new directions that better fit my goals or lifestyle?

At this stage, some pharmacists:

• Transition into leadership or administrative roles

• Move into consulting or industry positions

• Shift toward part-time or more flexible arrangements

• Reinvest in teaching, mentoring, or academic work

This is not stepping back.

It is recalibrating.

Residency and Advanced Training — **Strategic Decisions**

Residency is one of the most important early decisions in a Clinical Pharmacist's career.

• **PGY1** builds general clinical competence

• **PGY2** provides specialization

These programs:

- Increase access to competitive roles
- Strengthen clinical confidence
- Expand professional networks

But they also:

- Delay higher earnings
- Require additional time and energy

This decision should be made strategically—not automatically.

It should align with:

- Your career goals
- Your tolerance for delayed income
- The type of work you ultimately want to do

Board Certification and Continuing Education

Clinical pharmacy is a field that evolves continuously.

Staying current is not optional.

Common certifications include:

- Board Certified Pharmacotherapy Specialist (BCPS)
- Specialty certifications (oncology, ambulatory care, etc.)

In addition to certification, pharmacists are required to complete continuing education (CE) to maintain licensure.

This ensures:

- Ongoing competency
- Awareness of new medications and guidelines
- Professional credibility

But it also requires time, attention, and ongoing commitment.

Professional Organizations and Networking

Growth in this field is not just about knowledge.

It is also about connection.

Professional organizations offer:

- Continuing education opportunities
- Conferences and networking events
- Access to industry trends and research

- Career advancement pathways

Engaging in these communities can:

- Open doors to new roles
- Provide mentorship
- Keep you connected to the broader profession

Careers rarely grow in isolation.

The Role of Mentorship

Mentorship can accelerate your development in ways that experience alone cannot.

A strong mentor can help you:

- Navigate early career challenges
- Identify opportunities for growth
- Avoid common pitfalls
- Reflect on alignment and long-term goals

Mentorship does not have to be formal.

But it should be intentional.

Using Alignment to Guide Growth

At every stage of your career, Mason's Alignment Theory (MAT) remains relevant.

Using:

- **PACES™** (Personality, Aptitude, Constraints, Experience, Situation)
- **CARESET™** (Culture, Autonomy, Resources, Expectations, Environment, Team)

You can evaluate not just where you are—but where you are going.

Because growth without alignment can lead to:

- Increased stress
- Reduced satisfaction
- Long-term disengagement

While aligned growth creates:

- Sustainability
- Confidence
- A stronger sense of purpose

The Honest Takeaway

A Clinical Pharmacist career is not static.

It evolves.

And the people who build the most sustainable careers are not just those who work hard—

They are the ones who:

- Reflect regularly
- Adjust intentionally
- Stay aligned with who they are

There is no single "right" path.

But there is a path that fits you.

And the more thoughtfully you approach your development...

The more likely you are to build a career that not only succeeds—but lasts.

12

SIDE HUSTLES™

Income Streams, Flexibility, and Optionality for Clinical Pharmacists

For many Clinical Pharmacists, the primary role provides stability, structure, and a strong income.

But it does not always provide flexibility.

Or variety.

Or a sense of control over how—and where—you use your expertise.

That is where **Side Hustles™** come in.

Not as a replacement for your career.

But as a way to expand it.

To create additional income streams, explore new interests, and build optionality into your professional life.

Because one of the most powerful positions in any career is this:

You have choices.

Why Clinical Pharmacists Explore Side Hustles

Side hustles are not always about money.

They are often about alignment.

Clinical Pharmacists pursue additional income streams to:

- Reduce financial pressure (especially student loan debt)
- Create flexibility outside structured healthcare systems
- Explore interests beyond their primary role
- Build long-term exit or transition options
- Regain a sense of autonomy and control

For some, a side hustle becomes a meaningful extension of their work.

For others, it becomes a pathway to something entirely different.

Clinical-Adjacent Income Streams

These opportunities stay close to your core training and licensure.

They often require minimal retraining and allow you to leverage your existing expertise.

Medication Therapy Management (MTM):

Providing medication reviews and optimization services, often remotely or through contracted platforms.

Telepharmacy and Remote Verification:

Supporting medication verification or consultations in remote or underserved settings.

PRN or Per Diem Shifts:

Working additional hours in hospital or retail settings for supplemental income.

Immunization Clinics and Seasonal Work:

Participating in vaccination programs or public health initiatives.

These options tend to be the most straightforward to enter—and the easiest to scale up or down depending on your availability.

Non-Clinical and Consulting **Opportunities**

Some Clinical Pharmacists move beyond direct patient care into advisory or consulting roles.

These can include:

Pharmaceutical Writing and Medical Content Development:

Creating educational materials, drug information content, or clinical summaries.

Drug Information and Safety Consulting:

Supporting organizations with medication safety, formulary management, or clinical guidelines.

Expert Witness Work:

Providing professional insight in legal cases involving medication-related issues.

Healthcare Consulting:

Working with organizations to improve workflows, safety protocols, or clinical operations.

These paths often require strong communication skills and the ability to translate complex information into clear, actionable insights.

Digital and Scalable Income Streams

Technology has opened the door for pharmacists to build income streams that are not tied directly to hours worked.

Examples include:

Online Courses and Education Platforms:

Teaching topics related to pharmacology, exam preparation, or clinical practice.

Digital Products:

Creating templates, guides, or tools for students or professionals.

Content Creation (Blogs, Podcasts, Social Media):

Sharing expertise and building an audience over time.

Professional Branding and Thought Leadership:

Positioning yourself as an expert in a niche area.

These options often take longer to build—but can provide greater flexibility and scalability over time.

Academic and Teaching Roles

For those who enjoy education, teaching can be both rewarding and financially beneficial.

Options include:

Adjunct Faculty Positions:

Teaching part-time in pharmacy programs or healthcare courses.

Precepting Students:

Supporting the development of future pharmacists.

Continuing Education (CE) Development:

Creating or delivering educational content for licensed professionals.

These roles allow you to stay connected to the profession while contributing to its future.

Entrepreneurial Pathways

Some Clinical Pharmacists choose to build businesses based on their expertise.

Examples include:

- Specialty medication consulting services
- Compounding or niche pharmacy services
- Health coaching or medication adherence programs
- Private consulting or advisory practices

Entrepreneurship requires additional effort, risk tolerance, and business knowledge.

But it also offers the highest level of autonomy.

Important Considerations Before You Start

Side hustles can be valuable—but they require thoughtful planning.

Consider:

Time and Energy:

Do you have the capacity to take on additional work without burning out?

Conflict of Interest:

Does your employer allow outside work? Are there restrictions?

Licensure and Compliance:

Are there legal or regulatory requirements for the work you are considering?

Tax Implications:

Additional income may require planning for taxes and financial management.

Sustainability:

Is this something you can maintain long-term—or is it a short-term solution?

Not every opportunity is worth pursuing.

Alignment matters here, too.

The Role of Optionality

The true value of Side Hustles™ is not just additional income.

It is optionality.

It is knowing that:

- You are not limited to a single role
- You can adapt as your interests or circumstances change
- You have the ability to create new paths when needed

That kind of flexibility changes how you experience your primary career.

It reduces pressure.

And it increases confidence.

Alignment Still Comes First

Even when exploring additional income streams, Mason's Alignment Theory (MAT) still applies.

Using:

- **PACES™** (Personality, Aptitude, Constraints, Experience, Situation)
- **CARESET™** (Culture, Autonomy, Resources, Expectations, Environment, Team)

You can evaluate whether a side hustle:

- Fits your energy and interests
- Supports your long-term goals
- Enhances—not drains—your overall career

Because more work is not always better work.

The goal is not to do more.

It is to do what fits.

The Honest Takeaway

Clinical Pharmacists have more options than many people realize.

Beyond traditional roles, there are multiple ways to:

- Increase income
- Expand your skill set
- Create flexibility
- Build long-term career resilience

You do not have to use all of them.

But it helps to know they exist.

Because the strongest careers are not just built on what you do every day—

They are built on the options you have when things change.

13

WORK SETTING DEEP DIVE™

Where Clinical Pharmacists Actually Work

Choosing to become a Clinical Pharmacist is only part of the decision.

Where you practice will shape how that decision feels—every single day.

Two pharmacists with the same degree, similar training, and identical credentials can experience completely different careers based on their work setting. One may feel energized, aligned, and engaged. The other may feel overwhelmed, disconnected, or quietly burned out.

This is not about the profession itself.

It is about the environment in which that profession lives.

This section is designed to give you a clear, honest look at the most common pharmacy work settings—not just what they are, but what they feel like. The pace, the pressure, the interaction level, and the type of stress each environment creates.

Because choosing the right setting is often more important than choosing the right career.

. . .

Retail Pharmacy — High Volume, High Visibility, Constant Motion

Retail pharmacy is often the most visible and accessible form of pharmacy practice. It is where many pharmacists begin their careers, and where the public most frequently interacts with the profession.

The pace is fast, often driven by prescription volume, customer expectations, and operational demands. You may fill hundreds of prescriptions in a single shift, while also answering questions, administering vaccines, handling insurance issues, and managing workflow interruptions.

The stress here is not subtle.

It is immediate, constant, and tied to time pressure.

You are balancing accuracy with speed, often in an environment where interruptions are frequent and expectations are high. Patients are waiting, phones are ringing, and the line does not pause.

At the same time, retail offers something unique: **direct patient interaction.**

You build relationships. You answer questions in real time. You become a trusted resource in your community.

For some pharmacists, this is energizing.

For others, it becomes exhausting.

The key question is not whether retail pharmacy is "good" or "bad."

It is whether you thrive in an environment that is:

- Fast-paced
- Highly interactive
- Operationally intense
- Constantly moving

Hospital Inpatient Pharmacy — Structured, Clinical, Team-Based

Hospital inpatient pharmacy offers a different rhythm.

The environment is more structured, more clinically focused, and less driven by direct consumer interaction. Pharmacists review medication orders, verify dosing, monitor lab values, and collaborate with physicians and nurses to ensure safe and effective therapy.

The pace can still be demanding—but it is different.

Instead of customer-driven urgency, the pressure comes from **clinical responsibility.**

You are responsible for ensuring that every medication order is appropriate for the patient's condition. You are interpreting labs, identifying interactions, and preventing errors before they reach the patient.

The work requires sustained focus.

Long stretches of concentration. Continuous decision-making. Quiet accountability.

There is less interruption compared to retail—but more cognitive load.

For many pharmacists, this setting feels more aligned with why they entered the profession.

It offers:

- Clinical engagement
- Team collaboration
- Meaningful decision-making

But it also requires comfort with:

- Indirect patient interaction
- High responsibility
- Mental endurance

Intensive Care Unit (ICU) — **High Stakes, High Complexity**

The ICU is one of the most intense environments in healthcare.

Clinical Pharmacists in this setting manage medications for critically ill patients, often with rapidly changing conditions. Decisions are made quickly, and the margin for error is extremely small.

The pace is not always fast—but the **stakes are always high.**

You may spend significant time reviewing a single patient's regimen, ensuring every medication is appropriate, every dose is precise, and every interaction is considered.

This environment requires:

- Deep clinical knowledge
- Confidence in decision-making
- Comfort with uncertainty

Emotionally, it can be heavy.

You are working with patients who are unstable, sometimes at the edge of life. Outcomes are not always positive, despite your best efforts.

For some, this environment is deeply meaningful.

For others, it is overwhelming over time.

The alignment question here is simple:

Do you want to operate in a setting where every decision carries significant weight—and where that weight never fully goes away?

Ambulatory Care — **Relationship-Driven, Patient-Focused**

Ambulatory care pharmacists work in outpatient settings, often managing chronic conditions like diabetes, hypertension, or anticoagulation therapy.

This setting offers something many pharmacists seek:

Continuity.

You see patients over time. You adjust therapies. You track progress. You build relationships.

The pace is more predictable than retail or ICU settings, but the responsibility remains significant. You are often managing long-term treatment plans and helping patients navigate complex medication regimens.

Communication becomes a central skill.

You are not just verifying medications—you are explaining them, reinforcing adherence, and helping patients understand their role in their own care.

For pharmacists who value:

- Patient interaction
- Relationship building
- Ongoing care

this setting can feel highly aligned.

But it also requires patience, consistency, and the ability to manage long-term outcomes rather than immediate results.

Oncology Pharmacy — Precision, Emotion, and Responsibility

Oncology pharmacists work with cancer patients, managing chemotherapy and other complex therapies.

The level of precision required in this setting is extremely high.

Dosing must be exact. Timing matters. Small errors can have serious consequences.

But beyond the technical complexity, there is an emotional dimension.

You are working with patients facing life-altering diagnoses. You are part of a care team navigating uncertainty, hope, and difficult outcomes.

This setting requires:

- Technical accuracy
- Emotional resilience
- Strong communication

For some pharmacists, this is one of the most meaningful areas of practice.

For others, the emotional weight can be difficult to sustain over time.

Managed Care — Systems, Policy, and Population Health

Managed care pharmacists work behind the scenes, often within insurance companies or healthcare systems.

Their focus is not on individual prescriptions—but on **systems.**

They develop formularies, evaluate cost-effectiveness, and design policies that impact large populations.

The work is analytical and strategic.

You are using data to guide decisions, balancing clinical outcomes with financial considerations.

There is less direct patient interaction, but the impact is broad.

This setting is ideal for pharmacists who enjoy:

- Data analysis
- Systems thinking
- Policy development

It may feel less satisfying for those who prefer direct patient care.

Pharmaceutical Industry — Strategy, Science, and Scale

Pharmacists in the pharmaceutical industry work in areas like medical affairs, clinical research, and drug development.

The focus shifts from individual patients to **large-scale impact.**

You may be involved in:

- Clinical trials
- Drug safety monitoring
- Provider education

The work is often less repetitive and more project-based.

There is typically higher earning potential—but also different expectations, including travel, presentations, and performance metrics.

This setting appeals to pharmacists who enjoy:

- Communication
- Strategy
- Broad impact

It requires a shift in identity—from clinician to advisor or strategist.

Telepharmacy — Flexibility with Distance

Telepharmacy allows pharmacists to provide services remotely, using technology to verify prescriptions and consult with patients or providers.

This setting offers flexibility and can reduce some of the physical demands of traditional roles.

However, it also introduces:

- Reduced in-person interaction
- Dependence on technology
- Communication challenges

For some, this is a welcome shift.

For others, it may feel isolating.

The Alignment Question

Each of these settings is valid.

Each offers opportunities for impact.

But they are not interchangeable.

Using Mason's Alignment Theory (MAT), and applying:

- **PACES™**
- **CARESET™**

you can evaluate which environment fits you.

Because the same role can feel:

- Energizing in one setting
- Draining in another

The goal is not to find the "best" setting.

It is to find the one that fits you.

The Honest Takeaway

Pharmacy is not a single experience.

It is a collection of environments, each with its own pace, pressure, and personality.

Your degree gives you access.

Your choices determine your experience.

And the more clearly you understand these settings now—

The more intentional, aligned, and sustainable your career will be.

14

THE TRADEOFFS NO ONE EXPLAINS

What You Gain, What You Give, and Why It Matters

Every career is a tradeoff.

Not just in obvious ways like time and salary—but in the deeper, less visible ways that shape how you live your life over time.

Pharmacy is no exception.

In fact, because of the level of responsibility, precision, and consistency required, the tradeoffs in this profession are more pronounced than most people realize at the beginning.

And the sooner you understand them, the better your decisions become.

Because you are not just choosing a career.

You are choosing a pattern of living.

What You Gain — Stability, Structure, and Trust

One of the clearest advantages of pharmacy is stability.

You enter a profession where:

- your skills are consistently in demand
- your knowledge has real, immediate value
- your role is embedded in a system that depends on you

This creates a level of security that many careers cannot offer.

You are not guessing where you fit.

You are needed.

There is also structure.

Pharmacy is not a vague profession.

It is defined by:

- clear responsibilities
- established workflows
- measurable expectations

For many people, that structure is a strength.

It creates clarity.

It removes ambiguity.

It allows you to focus on execution rather than constantly redefining your role.

And then there is trust.

Once you establish yourself, people rely on you in ways that are significant.

Not casually.

Not occasionally.

Consistently.

Your decisions influence:

- medication safety
- patient outcomes
- team confidence

That level of trust is not given lightly.

And when it's earned, it becomes one of the most meaningful aspects of the work.

What You Give — Energy, Attention, and Consistency

But none of that comes without cost.

Pharmacy requires a specific type of output from you—every single day.

Not just effort.

But focused, disciplined, sustained attention.

You give:

- your concentration
- your mental energy

• your ability to stay precise even when you don't feel like it

And unlike some professions, you don't get to "dial it down" on certain days.

The expectation remains:

Be accurate.

Be alert.

Be responsible.

Even when:

• you're tired
• the workload is high
• the environment is chaotic

This consistency is what makes the role safe.

But it is also what makes it demanding.

The Tradeoff Most People Miss — Predictability vs. Flexibility

Pharmacy offers predictability.

You know:

• what the job requires
• how the workflow operates
• what success looks like

But that predictability often comes at the cost of flexibility.

Many roles involve:

• fixed schedules
• limited control over time off
• expectations that don't shift easily

Even in more flexible roles, the nature of the work itself requires presence.

You can't always:

• step away
• delay decisions
• shift responsibilities

Because the system depends on real-time accuracy.

For some people, this tradeoff works.

For others, it becomes a source of frustration.

The Emotional Tradeoff — Caring Without Closure

Pharmacy places you in a unique emotional position.

You are deeply connected to patient outcomes…

But not always directly connected to the patients themselves.

You may:

- adjust a therapy and never see the result
- prevent a complication without anyone realizing it
- contribute to a case without being part of the full story

This creates a form of emotional distance.

Not detachment.

But lack of closure.

You care.

You act.

But you don't always see the full impact.

For some, this is manageable.

For others, it creates a sense of incompleteness.

Understanding how you process that matters more than most people expect.

The Cognitive Tradeoff — Thinking as a Constant State

In pharmacy, thinking is not an occasional requirement.

It is the baseline.

You are always:

- evaluating
- verifying
- anticipating

Even when tasks appear routine.

There is no true "autopilot."

And that means your mind is engaged for the majority of your shift.

This is where fatigue builds—not physically, but mentally.

The tradeoff is this:

You develop strong analytical skills, precision, and judgment…

But you expend significant cognitive energy doing it.

Over time, how you manage that energy becomes one of the most important factors in sustainability.

The Identity Tradeoff — Professional vs. Personal Space

Pharmacy is a profession that can easily extend beyond your work hours.

Not in tasks.

But in mindset.

You may find yourself:

- thinking through cases after you leave
- questioning decisions at home
- carrying the responsibility with you

This is not constant.

But it is common.

And it creates a subtle overlap between your professional and personal space.

The tradeoff is this:

You develop a strong sense of responsibility and awareness...

But you must actively create separation to protect your personal life.

Otherwise, the role expands beyond its boundaries.

The Growth Tradeoff — Depth vs. Variety

Pharmacy allows for deep expertise.

You can:

- specialize
- refine your knowledge
- become highly skilled in specific areas

But that depth often comes at the expense of variety.

Many roles involve:

- similar workflows
- repeated processes
- consistent patterns

This is not a flaw.

It is part of the design.

But it means you must decide:

Do you value mastery and depth...

Or constant novelty and change?

Neither is better.

But one will fit you more naturally.

Why These Tradeoffs Matter

Most dissatisfaction in pharmacy does not come from the profession itself.

It comes from misunderstanding the tradeoffs.

If you expect:

- constant variety in a structured role
- high flexibility in a system-driven environment
- visible recognition in a behind-the-scenes position

You will feel friction.

Not because the job is wrong.

But because the expectations don't match the reality.

Clarity removes that friction.

Choosing With Awareness

When you understand the tradeoffs, your decisions become more intentional.

You stop asking:

👉 "Is this a good job?"

And start asking:

👉 "Is this a good fit for how I want to work and live?"

That shift is everything.

Because a job can be objectively strong...

And still not be right for you.

Adjusting the Tradeoffs Over Time

The most successful pharmacists are not the ones who found the perfect role immediately.

They are the ones who adjusted their tradeoffs over time.

They:

- moved into roles that matched their energy
- changed environments when needed
- refined their responsibilities

They didn't accept the tradeoffs as fixed.

They shaped them.

That's the difference between staying stuck...

and building a career that works.

The Long-Term Perspective

Over the course of a career, these tradeoffs compound.

Small mismatches become larger ones.

Small alignments become strengths.

The decisions you make early:

- where you work
- how you work
- what you prioritize

They don't just affect your next step.

They influence your trajectory.

That doesn't mean you have to get it perfect.

But it does mean awareness matters.

Final Thought

Pharmacy is a profession built on precision, responsibility, and consistency.

It offers stability, purpose, and impact.

But it asks for something in return.

Your attention.

Your discipline.

Your energy.

The goal is not to avoid that exchange.

It is to make sure it is one that works for you.

Because when the tradeoffs are aligned with who you are...

The work feels sustainable.

And when they're not...

Even a good career can feel like the wrong one.

15

THE FIRST FIVE YEARS™

What Your Early Career Actually Feels Like

The transition from pharmacy school to real-world practice is one of the most misunderstood phases of the profession.

Most people assume that once you graduate, pass your boards, and land your first job, the hard part is over.

In reality, the first five years of your career are where everything becomes real.

This is where knowledge meets responsibility.

Where confidence is built—or challenged.

Where alignment either strengthens... or begins to fracture.

This chapter is not about titles or promotions.

It is about what the experience actually feels like—year by year.

Year 0–1 — Shock, Responsibility, and Learning Under Pressure

Your first year as a pharmacist does not feel like mastery.

It feels like awareness.

You quickly realize that everything you learned in school was necessary—but not sufficient for the complexity of real-world practice. The safety nets feel thinner. The decisions feel heavier. And the realization that your judgment directly impacts patient outcomes becomes very real, very quickly.

There is a constant internal dialogue:

- Did I miss anything?
- Is this dose correct?
- Should I double-check that again?

Even routine tasks can feel intense because the stakes are no longer theoretical.

Confidence does not come immediately.

It builds slowly—through repetition, correction, and experience.

This year is less about being perfect and more about becoming reliable.

You learn your systems.

You learn your team.

You learn your own patterns under pressure.

And most importantly—you learn that being careful is not a weakness.

It is the foundation of the role.

Year 2–3 — Competence, Speed, and the Beginning of Fatigue

By your second and third years, something shifts.

You are no longer new.

You understand workflows. You recognize patterns. You move more quickly through your responsibilities. Tasks that once required intense focus begin to feel more familiar.

This is where **competence develops.**

But something else can begin to appear alongside it:

Fatigue.

Not from lack of ability—but from sustained cognitive effort.

You are still:

- Reviewing
- Verifying
- Evaluating

• Deciding

But now you are doing it faster, with higher expectations, and often with less external feedback.

This is also when many pharmacists begin to notice aspects of the role that either align—or don't.

You may find yourself thinking:

• I enjoy this part of the job

• This part drains me more than I expected

This is not failure.

It is clarity.

These years are where your professional identity begins to take shape.

Year 4–5 — Stability, Questions, and the Pivot Point

By years four and five, you are no longer developing basic competence.

You are established.

You understand your environment, your responsibilities, and your role within the system.

And this is where an important question begins to surface:

Do I want to keep doing this—exactly as it is?

For some pharmacists, the answer is yes.

They have found alignment. The work fits how they think, how they operate, and what they value.

For others, this is where the first real tension appears.

Not because they cannot do the job—but because sustaining it begins to feel heavier than expected.

This is the **pivot window**.

You may choose to:

• Specialize

• Change settings

• Reduce hours

• Explore non-clinical roles

Or you may choose to stay—and refine your environment.

There is no single right answer.

But this is the stage where intentional decisions matter most.

The Confidence Curve — **What No One Explains Clearly**

Confidence in pharmacy does not arrive all at once.

It builds unevenly.

Early on, confidence is fragile.

You second-guess decisions. You double-check constantly. You rely on protocols and confirmation.

Over time, confidence becomes more internal.

You recognize patterns faster. You trust your judgment more. You begin to operate with greater independence.

But even experienced pharmacists encounter moments of uncertainty.

And that is part of the role.

The goal is not to eliminate doubt.

It is to manage it—without letting it slow you down or compromise your decisions.

The Burnout Window — **When It Begins (and Why)**

Burnout in pharmacy rarely appears suddenly.

It builds.

Often during years two through five, when:

- Work becomes routine
- Expectations increase
- Feedback decreases
- Cognitive load remains constant

You may begin to feel:

- Mentally fatigued
- Less engaged
- More reactive to interruptions
- Less connected to the meaning behind the work

This is not a sign that you chose the wrong career.

It is a signal that something may need to adjust.

That adjustment could be:

- Environment
- Schedule
- Role type
- Or even expectations

Recognizing this early is critical.

The Salary vs. Stress Reality

One of the most common realizations during the first five years is the relationship between compensation and workload.

Pharmacy offers strong earning potential.

But that income is tied to:

- Responsibility
- Attention to detail
- Sustained mental effort

Many pharmacists reach a point where they ask:

Is the compensation aligned with how this work feels day to day?

For some, the answer is yes.

For others, it becomes a reason to explore different paths within the profession.

This is where financial understanding and alignment intersect.

Why Some Pharmacists Leave (and Others Stay)

Not everyone stays in the same role long-term.

Some pharmacists leave their initial setting within the first five years.

Common reasons include:

- Misalignment with workflow or pace
- Desire for more or less patient interaction
- Burnout or fatigue
- Interest in other opportunities

Others stay—and thrive.

Often because:

- The environment fits them
- The expectations match their strengths
- The work feels sustainable

The difference is rarely about ability.

It is about fit.

Using **Alignment to Guide Your Early Career**

This is where Mason's Alignment Theory (MAT) becomes practical.

Using:

- **PACES™**
- **CARESET™**

you can evaluate not just your role—but your experience within that role.

Ask yourself:

- Does this environment support how I think?
- Does this pace match my energy?
- Does this level of responsibility feel sustainable?

Small adjustments early can prevent larger problems later.

The Honest Takeaway

The first five years of a pharmacy career are not just about learning the job.

They are about learning yourself within the job.

You will:

- Build confidence
- Experience pressure
- Discover what fits—and what doesn't

And those discoveries matter more than any title.

Because the goal is not just to succeed early.

It is to build something you can sustain.

16

#1 DAY IN THE LIFE - HOSPITAL PHARMACIST

Name: Polly Pillcount, PharmD — "The Dose Defender"

Scrub Color: Violet Veil

Primary Role: Hospital Pharmacist (Acute Care / Inpatient)

This Role Also Aligns With: Clinical Pharmacist (PharmD); Medication Safety Officer (PharmD, MS); Pharmacy Operations Supervisor (PharmD, MBA)

SCRUBfit™ Category: Med Heads

Pros: High impact on patient safety; interdisciplinary collaboration; constant learning.

Cons: High responsibility; interruptions; rapid pace with little margin for error.

Personality Traits: Analytical, composed, compassionate, vigilant.

Clinical tools: BD Pyxis (gl), Epic (gl), Micromedex (gl), Alaris smart pump (gl), 3M badge reader, pill counter, communication board, barcode scanner.

Clinical Confession: "The moment I verify a high-alert med, I whisper 'safe passage.' It's my tiny ritual of care."

Character Description

Polly Pillcount moves through the quiet hum of the Central Pharmacy like an orchestra conductor tuned to a heartbeat. Her Violet Veil scrubs catch the light as she checks the morning queue of pending orders, eyes tracing the line items with deliberate calm. She's not just dispensing drugs—she's safeguarding stories. Every order represents someone's loved one, waiting upstairs under fluorescent light and hope.

Her calm precision anchors the team during chaos. When a crash cart tray is delayed or an override request pings from the ICU, Polly's instinct is both clinical and human—"What does the patient need right now, and what can't wait?" Her discipline is quiet but unshakeable. She carries the serenity of someone who knows that pharmacy isn't a supporting act; it's the silent foundation of safety.

Polly didn't always plan to work in a hospital. Retail had once seemed more personal—names, faces, families—but the lure of critical care drew her into the kinetic heartbeat of inpatient life. Here, she could see the science unfold in real time: vancomycin levels adjusting, anticoagulants fine-tuned, pain pumps recalibrated. She began to understand that stewardship isn't about speed; it's about precision in motion.

Day in the Life (06:45–18:30)

05:30 — Wake-Up.

Polly's alarm hums softly before sunrise, a gentle chime she chose specifically because it doesn't jolt her awake. For a moment, she lies still, listening—to the quiet of her townhouse, to the faint bubbling of the freshwater aquarium in the corner of her living room. Neon tetras glide through the plants in slow, rhythmic motion, a calm counterpoint to the pace of her day ahead.

She swings her feet onto the cool hardwood floor and stretches, already running through a mental checklist. ICU census was high yesterday. She wonders if any of those patients destabilized overnight. That thought lingers—not as anxiety, but as awareness.

05:40 — Morning Routine.

In the kitchen, she measures coffee grounds with the same precision she uses at work. Two scoops. No guesswork. The coffee maker hums to life as she opens the back door to let her golden retriever, Sunny, out into the early morning air.

"Quick one," she says softly. Sunny trots out, tail wagging, while Polly refills his water bowl and scoops kibble into his dish. She pauses for a moment, watching him eat. This is her quiet—her reset before stepping into a world where nothing is ever slow.

05:55 — Aquarium and Stillness.

Before getting dressed, she feeds the fish—just a pinch, careful not to overdo it. Even here, balance matters. Too much and the system gets unstable. Too little and something suffers. She smiles faintly at the parallel.

06:05 — Getting Ready.

Her Violet Veil scrubs are laid out from the night before. She dresses quickly, ties her hair back, and clips her badge onto her waistband. In the mirror, she takes a breath. Calm in. Focus out.

06:20 — Commute.

The drive to Hopewell Hospital is familiar—same turns, same traffic lights, same quiet stretch of road where the sun begins to rise just over the tree line. She keeps the radio low, not music, just background noise. Her mind is already shifting into clinical mode.

She replays common scenarios: renal dosing adjustments, anticoagulation checks, high-alert medications. It's not worry—it's preparation. By the time she pulls into the parking garage, she's already halfway into the role.

06:45 — Badge In.

The elevator doors open to the hum of Hopewell's Central Pharmacy. The day shift arrives with the scent of coffee and the whir of automated dispensers. Polly logs into Epic (gl), scanning overnight notes. Two pages of IV orders, a vancomycin trough (gl) pending, and a new admit flagged "sepsis—broad spectrum started."

07:10 — Morning Handoff.

The night pharmacist briefs the team: "ICU had a norepi (gl) par increase, one override—approved; peds oncology pending IV cyclophosphamide double-check." Polly notes the high-alerts and glances at the Feedback Flow Board (Green=Approved with go-live date; Yellow=Under Review; Red=Not Approved with reason). Today's yellow item: new PCA (gl) library updates for Max Volt's smart-pump testing.

07:45 — Verifications.

Orders stream through: cefepime, vancomycin, levothyroxine. Each click is a decision, a trust exercise. A resident types "stat morphine 2 mg IV push," and Polly calls upstairs. "Can you verify pain score and sedation level?" She knows no order exists in isolation. Behind every vial is a patient who deserves clarity.

09:30 — IV Room Check.

Polly steps into the cleanroom. The air hisses through HEPA filters. A tech draws lines of saline and antibiotic under the sterile hood. "Good catch on that amio concentration yesterday," she says. "Saved us a near-miss." The tech smiles. Small praise, big meaning.

10:45 — Bedside Consult.

She rounds with an internal medicine team—an attending, two residents, and a nurse practitioner. The topic: renal dosing for piperacillin-tazobactam. Polly reviews the patient's creatinine clearance and recalculates. "Let's switch to 3.375 grams q8h extended infusion," she advises. They nod. Decisions ripple outward—one recalibration, hundreds of lives safer each year.

12:15 — Lunch (Sort Of).

Her salad waits as she fields a call: "ED has a code stroke—alteplase (gl) ready?" "Yes, verify dose and grab kit 4B," she answers. She eats standing up, fork in one hand, phone in the other. In healthcare, hunger waits behind safety.

14:00 — Formulary Meeting.

Conference call with Pharmacy & Therapeutics. The agenda: shortage management for cefazolin, a new oncology drug approval, and an alert from ISMP (gl) on look-alike/sound-alike (gl) packaging. Polly advocates for staff education and enhanced barcode scanning. "Technology can't replace vigilance—it should reinforce it."

16:30 — Afternoon Sweep.

One new admit, one stat heparin drip, one discharge med reconciliation (gl) left. She messages the nurse: "Patient's INR (gl) therapeutic; resume home warfarin." Every task ties back to one invisible word: trust.

17:50 — End-of-Shift Rounds.

Polly signs out, updates the Feedback Flow Board, and leaves a note under "Bright Spots": "New barcode training rolled out—zero overrides today." She exhales, a small release of tension she didn't realize she was holding.

18:30 — Badge Out.

As the automatic doors slide shut, she hears the familiar hum fade behind her. The evening air feels different—lighter, quieter.

18:50 — Drive Home.

Traffic moves slower now. She doesn't turn on the radio. Her mind replays the day—not obsessively, just enough to close the loop. The morphine call. The IV check. The near-miss that never became a miss.

19:10 — Home Reset.

Sunny greets her at the door, tail thumping against the wall. She kneels to scratch behind his ears, the first real moment of stillness all day. In the living room, the aquarium glows softly. The fish move the same way they did this morning—steady, unaffected by the chaos she just left.

She feeds Sunny, changes out of her scrubs, and exhales fully for the first time.

Before heading to the kitchen, she glances once more at the tank. Balance restored. System stable.

She smiles.

Another day of safe passage.

Alignment Insight

Hospital pharmacy is where precision becomes compassion in motion. Polly's alignment thrives in structure and impact—seeing her knowledge translate into immediate safety. For her, success isn't applause; it's a full medication pass with zero errors and one grateful nurse who whispers, "Thanks for catching that." Alignment, she's learned, feels like confidence you can stand on.

17

#3 DAY IN THE LIFE DITL #3 — CLINICAL PHARMACIST (INTERNAL MEDICINE)

Name: Dr. Caden Chartwell, PharmD, BCPS — "The Clinical Compass"

Scrub Color: Graphite Gray

Primary Role: Clinical Pharmacist (Internal Medicine Service)

This Role Also Aligns With: Clinical Coordinator (PharmD, BCPS, MS); Residency Preceptor (PharmD, BCPS); Clinical Manager (PharmD, MBA)

SCRUBfit™ Category: Med Heads

Pros: Interprofessional respect; intellectual challenge; direct patient impact; teaching opportunities.

Cons: Documentation overload; time pressure; rounding fatigue; navigating team dynamics.

Personality Traits: Methodical, articulate, inquisitive, empathic.

Clinical tools: Epic (gl); UpToDate (gl); Micromedex (gl); clinical decision support dashboards; antibiotic stewardship tracker; patient handoff sheet; iPad for bedside reconciliation.

Clinical Confession: "I still triple-check vancomycin levels before rounds—because stewardship starts with humility."

Character Description

Dr. Caden Chartwell carries a quiet kind of authority—one that doesn't need volume to be felt. His Graphite Gray scrubs mirror his approach: steady, composed, grounded in clarity. He doesn't rush decisions, even when everything around him moves quickly. Instead, he slows the moment just enough to think, to question, to ensure that every recommendation is rooted in both evidence and intention.

He's known on the unit not just for what he knows, but how he teaches. When residents hesitate, he doesn't correct them outright. He asks, "What are you seeing?"—inviting them into the thinking process rather than shutting it down. His presence transforms uncertainty into learning.

For Caden, clinical pharmacy is not about being right—it's about being responsible. Every recommendation carries weight, even when it's delivered quietly. Especially then.

Day in the Life (06:45–18:30)

05:20 — Wake-Up.

Caden wakes before the alarm, the room still dim with early morning gray. For a moment, he stays still, listening—to the quiet hum of his apartment, to the low filtration sound of the saltwater aquarium across the room.

Inside the tank, a pair of clownfish drift between coral branches, slow and deliberate. It's the same environment he created for himself —controlled, balanced, intentional.

He exhales slowly, already aware of the day ahead. Not anxious. Not rushed. Just mentally stepping into motion.

05:30 — Morning Routine.

He moves through the apartment with quiet efficiency. Coffee starts first—measured, precise. While it brews, he checks overnight labs on his phone. Not required, but he prefers not to walk in blind.

Potassium drop. INR elevation. One flagged note for renal decline.

He nods slightly. "We'll adjust," he murmurs.

05:45 — Reset and Preparation.

He feeds the fish carefully, sprinkling just enough to keep the ecosystem stable. Too much throws everything off. Too little creates stress.

The parallel isn't lost on him.

Breakfast is simple—eggs, toast, black coffee. He eats sitting down, not rushed. This is his one intentional pause before the pace begins.

06:05 — Getting Ready.

Graphite Gray scrubs. Badge clipped. Watch set. Everything in place. He checks his bag—tablet, notes, backup pen. No wasted movement.

06:20 — Commute.

The drive is quiet. Early light filters through the windshield as the city slowly wakes. He doesn't play music. Instead, he reviews patient scenarios mentally.

Warfarin adjustment. Antibiotic de-escalation. Renal dosing.

Not memorization—preparation.

By the time he pulls into the hospital garage, he's already in clinical mode.

06:45 — Pre-Rounds.

Caden logs into Epic (gl), scanning overnight updates. Each patient is a story mid-sentence—he's responsible for reading what's already written and anticipating what comes next.

He writes quick notes on his handoff sheet:

"Hold warfarin."

"Recheck potassium."

"Monitor renal trend."

The floor begins to stir around him. Nurses moving. Monitors chiming. Breakfast trays rolling.

07:30 — Interdisciplinary Rounds.

The team gathers—attending, residents, nurses, case manager. They move room to room, decisions unfolding in real time.

"Cultures grew ESBL E. coli," a resident reports.

Caden steps in calmly. "Let's narrow from meropenem to ertapenem."

The attending nods. "Pharmacy-approved."

It's quick. Efficient. But the impact extends far beyond the moment.

09:15 — Medication Reconciliation.

A new patient sits quietly, a plastic bag filled with medication bottles in their lap.

Caden pulls up a chair, lowering himself to eye level. “Let’s go through these together,” he says.

One by one, they sort. Prescriptions. Supplements. Over-the-counter additions.

He catches an interaction with warfarin. Subtle. Easy to miss.

“Good catch,” the nurse says.

Caden nods once. For him, it’s not a moment—it’s the standard.

11:00 — Documentation Block.

Back at his workstation, he translates clinical thinking into documentation. Renal dosing adjustment. Antibiotic timing. Anticoagulation plan.

The work here is quiet, but it matters. What gets written becomes what gets followed.

12:30 — Teaching Moment.

A resident approaches, hesitant. “How do you decide when to restart anticoagulation after a GI bleed?”

Caden turns slightly, pulling up UpToDate (gl).

“Guidelines give you a range,” he says. “But the decision lives in the patient.”

The resident nods, thinking.

That’s the goal—not answers, but understanding.

14:00 — Rapid Response.

The call comes overhead. Urgency shifts instantly.

He moves quickly but without panic. Hypoglycemia case.

“Dextrose, 25 grams IV push,” he says, voice steady.

Numbers climb. Patient stabilizes.

The room exhales collectively.

Caden steps back quietly, already thinking through the follow-up.

15:45 — Family Conversation.

He sits with a patient’s daughter, explaining medication changes in clear, simple terms.

"We're reducing this to minimize side effects," he says. "Same goal, less burden."

She nods, relief visible.

This is the part that doesn't show up in documentation—but matters just as much.

17:15 — Wrap-Up and Mentorship.

He meets briefly with pharmacy residents, reviewing cases.

"What did you see today?" he asks.

Not what they did—what they understood.

They talk through decisions, adjustments, uncertainties.

Learning doesn't stop at rounds—it continues here.

18:30 — Badge Out.

Caden steps out of the hospital into evening light. The shift from constant noise to quiet is immediate.

18:50 — Drive Home.

The car is silent. He lets the day settle—not replaying everything, just enough to close it.

Decisions made. Risks reduced. Systems stabilized.

19:10 — Home Reset.

The aquarium glows softly in the dim room. The fish move the same way they did this morning—balanced, steady, unaffected by the complexity he just left.

He feeds them, washes his hands, and sits down for a moment without moving.

No alarms. No pages. No decisions.

Just stillness.

And the quiet understanding that clarity—applied consistently—changes outcomes.

Alignment Insight

Clinical pharmacy is alignment through inquiry. Caden thrives in the space between uncertainty and clarity—where thoughtful questions prevent silent harm. His alignment lives in the discipline of thinking deeply and acting deliberately. Success, to him, is not being seen—it's knowing that what he did mattered.

18

#4 DAY IN THE LIFE — ONCOLOGY PHARMACIST

Name: Dr. Isla IntraVen, PharmD, BCOP — "The Hope Compounder"

Scrub Color: Rose Quartz

Primary Role: Oncology Pharmacist (Inpatient & Infusion Center)

This Role Also Aligns With: Infusion Pharmacist (PharmD); Chemotherapy Safety Officer (PharmD, BCOP); Oncology Clinical Specialist (PharmD, BCOP, MS)

SCRUBfit™ Category: Med Heads

Pros: Deep patient relationships; precision-driven care; collaboration with oncologists and nurses; emotionally meaningful work.

Cons: Emotional fatigue; constant vigilance; drug shortages; long verification times.

Personality Traits: Gentle, meticulous, emotionally intelligent, resilient.

Clinical tools: Epic Beacon (gl); chemotherapy compounding robot (gl); infusion pump (gl); USP 797 (gl) cleanroom; hazardous drug cabinet; body-surface-area calculator; PPE kit.

Clinical Confession: "Every chemo dose I verify feels like a prayer measured in milligrams."

Character Description

Dr. Isla IntraVen moves through the oncology pharmacy with quiet reverence, her Rose Quartz scrubs a soft contrast to the sterile white of the cleanroom. To her, pharmacy here isn't about pills—it's about possibility. Every order represents someone's fight, someone's future, someone's still.

She understands that oncology pharmacy is not for the faint-hearted. The math is exacting, the drugs unforgiving, and the margin for error nonexistent. But what keeps her anchored is not the science alone—it's the humanity threaded through every interaction. A hand held a second longer. A conversation that softens fear. A moment where medicine becomes something more than protocol.

For Isla, this is where precision meets purpose.

Day in the Life (07:00–19:00)

05:15 — Wake-Up.

The alarm sounds softly, but Isla is already awake. The early morning light filters through sheer curtains, casting a muted glow across the room. She lies still for a moment, aware of the emotional weight the day may carry—not as dread, but as respect.

At the foot of the bed, her silver tabby cat, Luna, blinks slowly, stretching into the quiet. Isla exhales gently. "Another day," she whispers, more intention than statement.

05:25 — Morning Routine.

She moves into the kitchen, starting water for tea instead of coffee. Something steady, calming. While it heats, she checks her phone—not messages first, but patient flags from the oncology system.

Three new chemo orders. One dose adjustment. One flagged lab value.

She nods once. Not overwhelmed—prepared.

05:40 — Centering.

Before breakfast, she feeds Luna and stands for a moment by the window. No music. No noise. Just stillness.

This is deliberate. Oncology requires more than knowledge—it requires presence.

05:50 — Breakfast.

Oatmeal, fruit, tea. Simple. Predictable. She eats slowly, intentionally, knowing this may be the only calm stretch of the day.

06:10 — Getting Ready.

Rose Quartz scrubs. Hair secured. Minimal jewelry—nothing unnecessary. She checks her bag: notebook, ID, lip balm, backup pen.

Everything in oncology has purpose. Even preparation reflects that.

06:25 — Commute.

The drive is quiet, roads still mostly empty. She keeps the radio off, allowing space for mental preparation.

She reviews key considerations:

- BSA calculations
- Renal adjustments
- Antiemetic protocols
- Patient tolerance

Not memorizing—grounding herself in the rhythm of the work.

06:50 — Arrival Pause.

She sits in the car for a moment before stepping out. One breath in. One breath out.

Then she walks in.

07:00 — Badge In.

The oncology pharmacy hums softly under fluorescent light. Isla checks overnight reports—no adverse events, one renal adjustment, multiple pending verifications.

She ties her hair tighter, steps into position, and begins.

07:30 — Verification Block.

Orders populate the screen: carboplatin, paclitaxel, doxorubicin.

Each one requires full attention—height, weight, labs, organ function, prior cycles. She recalculates BSA manually even when the system provides it.

Trust—but verify. Always.

08:45 — Cleanroom Entry.

Inside the USP 797 (gl) cleanroom, everything slows down. The hum of filtration. The controlled airflow. The deliberate movements.

Technicians move with practiced precision. Isla oversees, checks, confirms.

"Cisplatin concentration verified," she says softly.

Every word carries weight here.

10:15 — Patient Interaction.

In the infusion center, a patient sits wrapped in a blanket, anxiety visible despite the calm environment.

Isla kneels beside her. "We adjusted your pre-medications," she explains gently. "This should help with nausea."

The patient nods, eyes softening.

In this moment, knowledge becomes comfort.

12:00 — Midday Pause (Brief).

She sits with the team for a few minutes—nurses, a dietitian, another pharmacist. Conversation is light, but shared understanding runs deep.

They all carry the same weight, just differently.

12:20 — Back to Flow.

Another order flags—lab values trending down. She recalculates dosing, communicates with the oncologist.

"Reduce by 25%," she suggests.

Approved. Adjusted. Safer.

14:00 — Clinical Review.

A complex case. Multiple drugs. Renal compromise.

She slows everything down, breaking it into pieces. Evaluating interactions. Assessing tolerability.

This is where her skill lives—not speed, but precision under pressure.

15:45 — Family Conversation.

A patient's spouse asks, "Is this working?"

Isla doesn't rush the answer. "We're adjusting to make it as effective—and as tolerable—as possible," she says.

Honest. Measured. Human.

17:00 — Critical Catch.

A dose discrepancy surfaces—small, but significant.

She recalculates. Confirms. Corrects.

No one else may ever know—but she does.

"Safe passage," she whispers.

18:15 — Final Sweep.

She reviews remaining orders, checks documentation, ensures everything aligns.

Nothing rushed. Nothing skipped.

19:00 — Badge Out.

The infusion center quiets as the last patients leave. Isla removes her protective gown slowly, deliberately.

19:20 — Drive Home.

The sky is darker now. She drives in silence, letting the day settle. Not every thought lingers—but the meaningful ones do.

19:40 — Home Reset.

Luna greets her at the door. Isla kneels, letting the contact ground her.

She changes, washes her hands longer than necessary—a habit, a ritual, a release.

For a moment, she sits without moving.

No calculations. No alerts. No decisions.

Just quiet.

And the quiet understanding that today, precision carried hope forward—one dose at a time.

Alignment Insight

Oncology pharmacy is alignment through empathy and precision. Isla thrives where science meets humanity—where every calculation carries emotional weight. Her alignment lives in the ability to hold both truth and compassion at the same time. Success, to her, is not just safe dosing—it's making the experience of treatment just a little more bearable.

19

#5 DAY IN THE LIFE — CRITICAL CARE PHARMACIST

Name: Dr. Jason Ventrix, PharmD, BCCCP — "The Pressure Stabilizer"

Scrub Color: Steel Blue

Primary Role: Critical Care Pharmacist (ICU)

This Role Also Aligns With: Emergency Medicine Pharmacist (PharmD, BCPS); Code Team Pharmacist (PharmD, BCCCP); Clinical Specialist (PharmD, BCCCP)

SCRUBfit™ Category: Med Heads

Pros: High-impact decision-making; real-time interventions; respected clinical role; intellectually stimulating.

Cons: High stress; rapid pace; life-and-death decisions; emotional intensity.

Personality Traits: Focused, decisive, resilient, calm under pressure.

Clinical tools: Epic (gl); ICU monitoring systems; infusion pumps (gl); vasopressor (gl) titration charts; code cart; ventilator interface (gl); point-of-care labs.

Clinical Confession: "You don't rise to the moment in the ICU—you fall to your level of preparation."

Character Description

Dr. Mason Ventrix moves through the ICU with quiet intensity, his Steel Blue scrubs blending into the controlled chaos around him. The environment is never still—monitors beep, alarms sound, conversations overlap—but within that noise, he finds clarity.

He doesn't chase urgency. He organizes it. Every decision is calculated, every adjustment deliberate. In a setting where seconds matter, he brings something rare—calm that doesn't slow things down, but sharpens them.

Critical care is not about being fearless. It's about functioning precisely in the presence of fear. And Mason has learned to do exactly that.

Day in the Life (06:30–18:45)

05:10 — Wake-Up.

The alarm hits once. Mason is already reaching for it before it sounds a second time. No hesitation. No lingering.

He sits up immediately, body already aligned with the day ahead. The room is dark, quiet, controlled. Exactly how he likes it.

05:15 — First Check-In.

He swings his legs out of bed and pauses for a moment—not to relax, but to orient. ICU days don't start when you walk in—they start here, mentally.

In the corner, his Doberman, Atlas, lifts his head slightly, watching him with quiet alertness. "You're coming," Mason says. Atlas stands instantly.

05:20 — Movement.

They step outside into the cool morning air. Mason walks with purpose, Atlas at his side. No phone. No distractions. Just movement.

This is his only reset before stepping into intensity.

05:35 — Fuel.

Back inside, coffee starts immediately. Eggs, toast, nothing complicated. He eats sitting down, but quickly. Efficiency matters—but so does preparation.

He checks overnight ICU summaries on his phone. One intubation. One vasopressor escalation. One renal decline.

He nods once. "Alright."

05:50 — Getting Ready.

Steel Blue scrubs. Watch secured. Badge clipped. Everything has a place. Everything is functional.

He grabs his bag—tablet, notes, backup pen. Redundancy is not optional in critical care.

06:05 — Commute.

The drive is quiet, streets still waking up. Mason doesn't use music. His mind is already running simulations:

- Hypotension management
- Sedation adjustments
- Antibiotic coverage
- Electrolyte correction

He's not predicting the day—he's preparing for variability.

06:25 — Arrival Pause.

He parks, sits for five seconds, and inhales deeply. Not calm—focus.

Then he steps out.

06:30 — ICU Entry.

The unit is already alive. Monitors beeping. Ventilators cycling. Staff moving quickly.

Mason logs into Epic (gl) immediately, scanning overnight changes. Each patient is unstable in a different way. Each requires a different strategy.

07:00 — Pre-Rounds Assessment.

He builds his mental map:

Patient 1 — septic shock, escalating pressors

Patient 2 — post-op, unstable BP

Patient 3 — renal failure, electrolyte imbalance

No single problem. Multiple systems. Simultaneously.

07:30 — ICU Rounds.

The team moves fast—attending, residents, nurses.

"MAP dropping to 60," a nurse reports.

Mason responds instantly. "Increase norepinephrine by 2 mcg/min. Reassess in 5."

No hesitation. No overthinking. Just execution.

09:15 — Code Blue.

The overhead call cuts through everything.

Mason is already moving.

Inside the room, it's controlled chaos—compressions, voices, urgency.

"Epinephrine ready," he says, handing it off precisely.

Time compresses. Focus sharpens.

Then—pulse returns.

The room exhales.

Mason steps back, already thinking through next steps.

11:00 — Stabilization Phase.

Back on the unit, he reviews sedation levels, ventilator settings, vasopressor titrations.

This is the quieter part—but no less critical.

Small adjustments now prevent bigger crises later.

12:30 — Quick Break.

He sits briefly, protein bar in hand. No full meal. No downtime.

Just enough to reset.

13:00 — Clinical Deep Dive.

A complex patient requires full review—multiple medications, declining organ function.

Mason slows down, analyzing every variable.

This is where experience shows—not speed, but depth.

15:15 — Nurse Collaboration.

A nurse approaches with concern about a patient's sedation level.

Mason listens fully, then adjusts the plan.

Collaboration is constant—but so is trust.

16:45 — Late-Day Pressure.

Another instability. Blood pressure dropping again.

He adjusts quickly, communicates clearly.

No panic. Just precision.

17:45 — Final Review.

He walks through each patient one last time. Verifies plans. Confirms orders.

No loose ends.

18:45 — Badge Out.

The ICU hum fades as he steps out.

19:05 — Drive Home.

Silence. No replay. Just release.

19:25 — Home Reset.

Atlas greets him instantly, energy contained but ready.

Mason kneels, grounding himself in the moment.

Shoes off. Scrubs off.

He sits for a moment, still.

No alarms. No urgency.

Just quiet.

And the understanding that today, control existed where chaos tried to take over.

Alignment Insight

Critical care pharmacy is alignment under pressure. Mason thrives in environments where decisions must be made quickly and precisely. His alignment lives in control, preparation, and the ability to stabilize what others cannot. Success is not comfort—it's competence in the moments that matter most.

20

#6 DAY IN THE LIFE — EMERGENCY DEPARTMENT PHARMACIST

Name: Dr. Lila Statton, PharmD, BCPS — "The Rapid Responder"

Scrub Color: Crimson Pulse

Primary Role: Emergency Department Pharmacist

This Role Also Aligns With: Critical Care Pharmacist (PharmD, BCCCP); Trauma Pharmacist (PharmD, BCPS); Code Team Pharmacist (PharmD)

SCRUBfit™ Category: Med Heads

Pros: Immediate impact; dynamic environment; high clinical involvement; fast decision-making.

Cons: Unpredictable pace; emotional intensity; frequent interruptions; high stress.

Personality Traits: Quick-thinking, composed, assertive, adaptable.

Clinical tools: Epic ASAP (gl); code cart; automated dispensing cabinet (gl); point-of-care testing devices; rapid sequence intubation kit; trauma protocol sheets.

Clinical Confession: "In the ED, you don't get perfect information—you get seconds. You learn to trust your training."

Character Description

Dr. Lila Statton thrives in motion. In the Emergency Department, stillness doesn't exist—only brief pauses between waves. Her Crimson Pulse scrubs seem to match the tempo around her, moving quickly but never frantically.

She has a presence that cuts through noise. When voices rise, she lowers hers. When things speed up, she becomes more precise. It's not about controlling chaos—it's about navigating it without losing clarity.

For Lila, every moment matters because every patient arrives at a turning point. The ED isn't where stories begin—it's where they change direction. And she stands right at that pivot.

Day in the Life (07:00–19:30)

05:30 — Wake-Up.

The alarm vibrates softly against the nightstand. Lila reaches over and silences it before the second buzz. Her eyes open immediately, adjusting to the dim early morning light filtering through the blinds.

For a moment, she stays still—not resting, but orienting. Emergency medicine doesn't allow for slow starts.

At the edge of the bed, her mixed-breed rescue dog, Nova, lifts her head, ears perked. "You're up too?" Lila murmurs, swinging her legs over the side.

05:35 — First Movement.

They step outside into the quiet morning air. Nova moves ahead, alert and curious, while Lila walks with a steady pace, letting the cool air settle her mind.

No phone. No distractions. Just a brief moment of calm before unpredictability takes over.

05:50 — Kitchen Routine.

Coffee starts immediately. Strong. No hesitation.

She moves through the kitchen efficiently—feeding Nova, filling her water bowl, grabbing a quick breakfast. Eggs, toast, a few bites standing at the counter.

Her mind is already shifting: trauma alerts, stroke calls, overdose cases, unknowns. Always unknowns.

06:05 — Early Check-In.

She glances at her phone. Overnight notes from the ED team: two critical admits, one overdose stabilized, one pending psych transfer.

She nods once. That's enough context. The rest will unfold in real time.

06:15 — Getting Ready.

Crimson Pulse scrubs. Hair pulled tight. Badge clipped. Shoes laced firmly—she'll be moving nonstop.

She checks her bag—water bottle, snack, extra pen. No assumptions about breaks.

06:25 — Commute.

The roads are already building with early traffic. Lila merges confidently, eyes scanning constantly.

She doesn't play music. Instead, she runs through rapid-response scenarios in her head:

- Anaphylaxis
- Stroke protocol
- Rapid sequence intubation
- Pediatric dosing

She's not memorizing—she's priming.

06:50 — Parking Lot Pause.

She sits in the car for a moment, hands resting lightly on the steering wheel. One breath in. One breath out.

Then she steps into motion.

07:00 — ED Entry.

The Emergency Department is already alive. Monitors beep. Conversations overlap. Movement never stops.

Lila logs into Epic ASAP (gl), scanning the board. Patients line every column—some stable, some not.

There is no slow start.

07:20 — First Call.

"Possible stroke arriving in five."

Lila moves immediately, pulling up dosing protocols, checking weight estimates, preparing alteplase (gl).

When the patient arrives, everything accelerates.

"Time last known well?" she asks.

Information comes in fragments. She assembles it quickly.

Decision made. Medication prepared.

Time matters.

08:45 — Flow State.

The ED fills rapidly. Chest pain. Falls. Shortness of breath. Unknown complaints that could be anything—or everything.

Lila moves between stations, verifying orders, answering questions, anticipating needs.

A nurse calls out, "Can you check this dose?"

She's already there.

10:30 — Overdose Case.

A patient arrives unresponsive. Suspected opioid overdose.

"Naloxone ready," Lila says, drawing it up with practiced speed.

Moments later, the patient gasps awake.

The room shifts instantly—from crisis to stabilization.

Lila steps back, already thinking through next steps.

12:00 — Midday Compression.

There's no true break—just a brief pause between surges.

She leans against the counter, takes a sip of water, scans the board again.

New patients. New variables.

No reset—just continuation.

13:30 — Trauma Alert.

"Trauma incoming."

The energy changes immediately. Staff move faster, voices sharpen.

Lila positions herself near the code cart, reviewing medication protocols mentally.

When the patient arrives, it's controlled chaos—blood, movement, urgency.

"Epinephrine ready," she says, voice steady.

Everything happens quickly—but with purpose.

15:15 — Collaboration Moment.

A resident hesitates over an antibiotic choice.

Lila steps in calmly. “Let’s broaden coverage—then we can narrow once cultures return.”

The resident nods, confidence restored.

Teaching happens in seconds here—but it matters.

16:45 — Fatigue Edge.

The pace doesn’t slow—but the body feels it.

Lila rolls her shoulders slightly, resets her posture. Focus doesn’t drop—it sharpens.

This is where discipline matters most.

18:00 — Final Push.

The last wave hits. Patients waiting. Orders stacking.

She moves efficiently, prioritizing without hesitation.

No wasted motion. No unnecessary delay.

19:30 — Shift End.

The ED doesn’t stop—but her shift does.

She signs out quickly, ensuring continuity.

Then she steps out.

19:50 — Drive Home.

Silence fills the car. No radio. No replay.

Just decompression.

20:10 — Home Reset.

Nova greets her at the door, energy contained but present.

Lila kneels, grounding herself in the moment.

Shoes off. Scrubs off.

She sits for a moment without moving.

No alarms. No urgency. No unknowns.

Just stillness.

And the quiet understanding that in a place defined by uncertainty, she brought clarity—one decision at a time.

Alignment Insight

Emergency pharmacy is alignment in motion. Lila thrives where unpredictability meets preparation—where rapid decisions carry immediate consequences. Her alignment lives in speed, clarity, and composure under pressure. Success isn’t measured in calm days—it’s measured in controlled ones.

21

#7 DAY IN THE LIFE — AMBULATORY CARE PHARMACIST

Name: Dr. Elias Roundwell, PharmD, BCACP — "The Continuity Builder"

Scrub Color: Evergreen Calm

Primary Role: Ambulatory Care Pharmacist (Chronic Disease Management Clinic)

This Role Also Aligns With: Primary Care Clinical Pharmacist (PharmD, BCACP); Population Health Pharmacist (PharmD, MPH); Medication Therapy Management Specialist (PharmD)

SCRUBfit™ Category: Med Heads

Pros: Long-term patient relationships; structured schedule; measurable outcomes; collaborative care.

Cons: Repetitive workflows; documentation burden; slower pace; insurance barriers.

Personality Traits: Patient, communicative, detail-oriented, relationship-driven.

Clinical tools: Epic Ambulatory (gl); population health dashboards; A1C tracker (gl); blood pressure logs; medication reconciliation tools; telehealth platform.

Clinical Confession: "In ambulatory care, progress isn't dramatic —it's steady. And steady is what keeps people alive."

Character Description

Dr. Elias Roundwell moves through the clinic with a sense of continuity that contrasts sharply with the urgency of inpatient care. His Evergreen Calm scrubs reflect his approach—steady, grounded, and focused on long-term outcomes rather than immediate intervention.

He sees what others don't always notice—the slow patterns, the incremental changes, the habits that shape health over months and years. Where others react to crises, Elias works to prevent them.

For him, success is not measured in moments, but in trajectories. A lower A1C. A stabilized blood pressure. A patient who finally understands their medications. These are quiet wins—but they are lasting ones.

Day in the Life (08:00–17:30)

06:10 — Wake-Up.

Elias wakes to the soft tone of his alarm, the room already touched by early morning light. He doesn't rush. He sits up slowly, taking a moment to orient himself before stepping into the day.

At the foot of the bed, his beagle, Penny, thumps her tail gently against the blanket, already awake and waiting. "I know," he says softly. "We're getting up."

06:15 — Morning Routine.

He moves into the kitchen, starting coffee while Penny circles expectantly. He measures the grounds carefully, more out of habit than necessity.

Breakfast is simple—oatmeal, fruit, coffee. He eats at the table, not standing, not rushed. This is part of his rhythm—starting the day steady so it stays steady.

06:30 — First Walk.

Outside, the air is cool and quiet. Penny moves slowly, nose to the ground, while Elias walks without urgency.

This is his reset. No phone. No email. Just movement and space before the day begins.

06:50 — Planning Ahead.

Back inside, he checks his schedule. Full clinic day: diabetes follow-ups, hypertension management, one new patient consult.

He reviews notes briefly—not to memorize, but to reconnect. These aren't cases. They're people he knows.

07:10 — Getting Ready.

Evergreen Calm scrubs. Hair neat. Badge clipped. He packs his bag—tablet, notes, water bottle.

Everything about his preparation is deliberate, but unhurried.

07:30 — Commute.

Traffic builds gradually, but Elias doesn't react to it. He listens to soft music, something consistent and unobtrusive.

His mind shifts gently into clinical mode—reviewing goals, not crises. Adjustments, not emergencies.

07:55 — Arrival.

He parks, gathers his things, and walks into the clinic with the same steady pace. No pause needed. No mental reset required. He's already there.

08:00 — Clinic Opens.

He logs into Epic Ambulatory (gl), reviewing patient charts for the morning. Lab trends. Medication adherence. Previous notes.

He updates his mental framework for each patient—not starting from scratch, but continuing a story already in motion.

08:30 — First Patient.

A long-term diabetic patient sits across from him, glucose logs in hand.

Elias reviews them carefully. "You've been more consistent," he says.

The patient nods. Small progress—but meaningful.

They adjust insulin dosing slightly. Not a dramatic change—just enough to keep things moving in the right direction.

09:45 — Hypertension Follow-Up.

Another patient, another pattern. Blood pressure trending down, but not quite controlled.

Elias asks questions beyond the numbers. Diet. Stress. Sleep.

The answer isn't always in the medication—it's in the context.

11:00 — Documentation Flow.

He enters notes methodically. Clear. Structured. Actionable.

Documentation isn't an afterthought—it's continuity. What he writes now shapes what happens next.

12:15 — Lunch Break.

He sits outside with his lunch, a simple sandwich and fruit. No rushing. No multitasking.

This is intentional. The pace of his work allows for this—and he protects it.

13:00 — New Patient Consult.

A new patient arrives with multiple medications, unclear instructions, and visible confusion.

Elias slows everything down. One medication at a time. One explanation at a time.

Understanding builds gradually. Confidence follows.

14:30 — Telehealth Visit.

Through the screen, another patient checks in. Blood pressure readings. Medication adherence. Questions.

Even remotely, the connection is real.

Elias listens carefully, responding with clarity and patience.

16:00 — Late-Day Review.

He reviews outstanding notes, checks follow-ups, updates care plans.

No rush. No backlog. Just completion.

17:30 — End of Day.

He logs out, closes his notes, and stands up slowly. The clinic quiets as the day ends.

17:50 — Drive Home.

Traffic again, but steady. He listens to music, letting the day settle.

No replay needed. Progress was made. That's enough.

18:10 — Home Reset.

Penny greets him enthusiastically, tail wagging in full force. He kneels, grounding himself in the moment.

Shoes off. Scrubs off.

He sits for a moment, letting the quiet settle around him.

No urgency. No alarms.

Just steadiness.

And the quiet understanding that today, small changes moved lives forward.

Alignment Insight

Ambulatory care pharmacy is alignment through continuity. Elias thrives in environments where progress is gradual but meaningful. His alignment lives in relationships, patterns, and long-term outcomes. Success isn't dramatic—it's sustained.

22

#8 DAY IN THE LIFE — INFECTIOUS DISEASE PHARMACIST

Name: Dr. Rowan Clearwell, PharmD, BCIDP — "The Resistance Strategist"

Scrub Color: Deep Teal

Primary Role: Infectious Disease Pharmacist (Antimicrobial Stewardship)

This Role Also Aligns With: Clinical Pharmacist (PharmD, BCPS); Antibiotic Stewardship Coordinator (PharmD, BCIDP); Epidemiology Pharmacist (PharmD, MPH)

SCRUBfit™ Category: Med Heads

Pros: High clinical impact; intellectual challenge; system-wide influence; collaboration with specialists.

Cons: Constant vigilance; evolving pathogens; data-heavy work; delayed gratification.

Personality Traits: Analytical, strategic, detail-driven, quietly assertive.

Clinical tools: Epic (gl); antimicrobial stewardship dashboard; culture and sensitivity reports; antibiogram (gl); Micromedex (gl); infection control protocols; secure messaging system.

Clinical Confession: "You don't always see resistance forming—but you feel it when it's too late."

Character Description

Dr. Rowan Clearwell operates in a world where the enemy is often invisible. His Deep Teal scrubs blend into the hospital environment, but his focus is always one step ahead—tracking patterns, anticipating resistance, and adjusting therapy before problems surface.

He is not driven by urgency in the traditional sense. Instead, he works with a long view, understanding that every antibiotic decision today influences outcomes weeks, months, and even years from now.

For Rowan, the work is less about reacting and more about preventing—quietly shaping the trajectory of care through decisions that most people will never notice.

Day in the Life (07:30–18:15)

05:40 — Wake-Up.

Rowan wakes to a soft alarm, the room still dim and quiet. He opens his eyes slowly, taking a moment before moving. His mind doesn't rush—it organizes.

Across the room, his saltwater reef tank glows faintly under automated lighting. Coral sways gently, fish moving in slow, deliberate patterns. Balance, he thinks. Always balance.

05:50 — Morning Routine.

He moves into the kitchen, starting coffee while the room gradually fills with light. No phone yet. No data. Just routine.

He feeds the reef tank carefully, measuring the amount with precision. Too much disrupts the ecosystem. Too little creates imbalance. The parallel to his work is constant—and intentional.

06:05 — First Check-In.

Coffee in hand, he opens his tablet. Culture reports populate the screen.

MRSA flagged. E. coli sensitivities updated. One resistant strain trending upward.

He leans forward slightly, focus sharpening. This is where his day begins—not with patients, but with patterns.

06:20 — Breakfast.

Simple. Eggs, toast, black coffee. He eats seated, reviewing notes from the previous day. Adjustments made. Outcomes pending.

In infectious disease, feedback is rarely immediate. Decisions echo forward.

06:40 — Getting Ready.

Deep Teal scrubs. Badge secured. Tablet packed. Notes organized.

Everything about his preparation reflects his mindset—structured, intentional, precise.

07:00 — Commute.

The drive is quiet. Rowan doesn't use music. Instead, he reviews microbial patterns mentally, connecting data points from the morning reports.

He's not thinking about individuals yet—he's thinking about systems.

07:25 — Arrival Pause.

He sits briefly in the car, reviewing one last note. Resistant strain cluster on one unit.

He exhales once.

Then steps out.

07:30 — System Review.

Logged into Epic (gl), Rowan pulls up the antimicrobial stewardship dashboard.

Antibiotic usage trends. Resistance patterns. Active cultures.

He scans quickly, identifying anomalies. One unit stands out—higher broad-spectrum usage than expected.

That's where he starts.

08:15 — Targeted Intervention.

He reviews patient charts from that unit. Multiple patients on broad-spectrum antibiotics without clear de-escalation plans.

He sends secure messages to the care teams:

"Consider narrowing based on sensitivities."

"Review duration—therapy may be extended beyond necessity."

No confrontation. Just guidance.

09:45 — Rounds with ID Team.

He joins the infectious disease physicians, moving through patient cases.

"Cultures show susceptibility," Rowan says. "We can step down therapy."

The physician nods. "Agreed."

Small adjustment. System-wide impact.

11:30 — Data Deep Dive.

Back at his workstation, Rowan analyzes trends. Antibiotic usage, resistance shifts, compliance patterns.

This is his core work—not visible, but critical.

Patterns emerge only if you look closely enough.

12:45 — Lunch.

He eats quietly, reviewing notes. No rush, but no full disengagement either.

In this field, awareness doesn't turn off.

13:30 — Consult Call.

A physician calls about a complex infection case.

"Given the resistance profile, I'd recommend switching to..." Rowan explains, walking through the reasoning step by step.

Clarity replaces uncertainty.

15:00 — Infection Control Check-In.

He meets briefly with infection prevention staff. Discussion centers on trends, containment strategies, and education needs.

This is where individual decisions connect to institutional outcomes.

16:30 — Follow-Up Loop.

Rowan revisits earlier recommendations. Some accepted. Some pending.

He adjusts where needed, reinforcing where appropriate.

Stewardship is persistence, not one-time action.

17:30 — Final Review.

He scans the dashboard one last time. No new alerts. No immediate concerns.

For him, that's success—problems prevented before they escalate.

18:15 — Badge Out.

He steps out of the hospital into the evening air, the shift from data to quiet immediate.

18:35 — Drive Home.

The car is silent. He doesn't replay the day—he reflects on patterns.

What shifted. What didn't. What needs attention tomorrow.

18:55 — Home Reset.

The reef tank glows again, more vibrant now under evening light. Rowan pauses in front of it, watching the movement.

He feeds the fish carefully, maintaining balance.

Shoes off. Scrubs off.

He sits for a moment, letting the quiet settle fully.

No alerts. No data streams.

Just stillness.

And the quiet understanding that today, unseen decisions shaped safer outcomes.

Alignment Insight

Infectious disease pharmacy is alignment through foresight. Rowan thrives in systems thinking, where patterns matter more than moments. His alignment lives in prevention, strategy, and quiet influence. Success isn't visible—it's the absence of problems that never had a chance to grow.

23

#9 DAY IN THE LIFE — PEDIATRIC PHARMACIST

Name: Dr. Nora Littlewell, PharmD, BCPPS — "The Gentle Calculator"

Scrub Color: Soft Sky Blue

Primary Role: Pediatric Clinical Pharmacist (Inpatient)

This Role Also Aligns With: Neonatal Pharmacist (PharmD, BCPPS); Pediatric Oncology Pharmacist (PharmD, BCPPS); Pediatric Medication Safety Specialist (PharmD)

SCRUBfit™ Category: Med Heads

Pros: Meaningful impact on vulnerable patients; strong team collaboration; highly specialized care; emotionally rewarding.

Cons: High emotional weight; zero margin for dosing error; parental anxiety; constant vigilance.

Personality Traits: Compassionate, meticulous, patient, emotionally attuned.

Clinical tools: Epic (gl); weight-based dosing calculator; pediatric dosing charts; syringe pump (gl); barcode medication administration system (gl); neonatal dosing references.

Clinical Confession: "In pediatrics, every decimal point feels like it matters more—because it does."

Character Description

Dr. Nora Littlewell carries a quiet gentleness into every room she enters, her Soft Sky Blue scrubs reflecting the calm she works so hard to maintain. In pediatric pharmacy, the margin for error is smaller, the stakes feel heavier, and the emotional weight lingers longer.

She understands that she is not only caring for patients—she is caring for families. Every explanation, every reassurance, every calculation carries an added layer of responsibility.

For Nora, precision is not just clinical—it is compassionate. Getting it right is how she protects both the child and the trust placed in her.

Day in the Life (07:00–18:15)

05:35 — Wake-Up.

Nora's alarm chimes softly, a gentle sound chosen on purpose. She opens her eyes slowly, letting herself wake gradually rather than abruptly. Pediatric days require calm from the very beginning.

Beside her bed, her small Cavalier King Charles Spaniel, Daisy, stirs and stretches, tail wagging lightly against the blanket. Nora smiles faintly. "Good morning, sweet girl."

05:40 — First Moments.

She sits up slowly, taking a breath before standing. The apartment is quiet, wrapped in early morning stillness.

This quiet matters. It's the last uninterrupted space before stepping into a world that requires constant attention.

05:45 — Morning Routine.

In the kitchen, Nora starts water for tea. Coffee feels too sharp for the kind of day she needs to have.

She feeds Daisy, watching her eat with content focus. That small normalcy grounds her.

Breakfast is light—toast, fruit, tea. She eats sitting down, unhurried, letting herself remain steady before the day begins to pull at her attention.

06:00 — Mental Preparation.

She checks her phone for overnight pediatric unit updates.

One NICU admission. One medication adjustment flagged. One note about feeding intolerance.

Her expression softens slightly. These are not just cases—they are tiny lives, fragile and evolving.

06:15 — Getting Ready.

Soft Sky Blue scrubs. Hair pulled back neatly. Minimal jewelry.

She checks her bag carefully—notes, tablet, extra pen. Pediatric work requires precision, and preparation supports that.

06:30 — Commute.

The drive is quiet, the early light soft across the road. Nora keeps the radio off.

Instead, she mentally reviews dosing considerations: weight-based calculations, concentration adjustments, infusion rates.

In pediatrics, everything is scaled—and everything must be exact.

06:55 — Arrival Pause.

She parks and sits for a moment, hands resting in her lap. One breath in. One breath out.

Then she steps into motion.

07:00 — Pediatric Unit Entry.

The floor is quieter than adult units, but the intensity is different. Monitors beep softly. Nurses move carefully. Parents sit close to bedsides.

Nora logs into Epic (gl), reviewing overnight notes. Each patient is small—but the complexity is not.

07:30 — First Review.

She begins with medication orders, double-checking weight-based dosing calculations.

A decimal point stands out—slightly off.

She recalculates. Confirms. Adjusts.

No one else may notice—but she does.

08:45 — NICU Consult.

A premature infant requires medication adjustment.

Nora reviews weight, gestational age, renal function—every variable matters.

She speaks quietly with the neonatologist, explaining her recommendation.

The plan changes—slightly, but safely.

10:15 — Parent Interaction.

A parent approaches, worry visible.

"Can you explain what this medication does?" they ask.

Nora kneels slightly, lowering herself to their level.

"It helps support their breathing," she explains gently, choosing words carefully.

Understanding replaces fear, even if only partially.

12:00 — Midday Pause.

She steps into the break room briefly, sipping tea. No full disengagement—just enough to reset her focus.

The emotional weight doesn't leave—it softens.

12:30 — Medication Preparation Oversight.

She reviews compounded pediatric medications, ensuring accuracy in concentration and labeling.

Everything must be exact. There is no tolerance for approximation here.

14:00 — Clinical Collaboration.

The team discusses a complex pediatric case. Multiple medications, evolving condition.

Nora listens fully before speaking.

"Let's adjust the dose slightly based on weight change," she suggests.

The team agrees.

Small adjustment. Significant impact.

15:45 — Emotional Moment.

A child begins to cry during medication administration.

Nora steps closer, voice soft, presence calm.

"It's okay," she says gently, more for the parent than the child.

Compassion is part of the protocol here.

17:00 — Final Checks.

She reviews all remaining orders, ensuring nothing is missed.

Fatigue is present—but precision remains.

17:45 — End-of-Day Review.

She updates notes, confirms plans, prepares for handoff.

Every detail matters—especially at transition points.

18:15 — Badge Out.

She steps out quietly, the shift from emotional intensity to silence immediate.

18:35 — Drive Home.

The car is quiet. Nora doesn't replay everything—but certain moments linger.

A parent's question. A child's cry. A safe adjustment.

18:55 — Home Reset.

Daisy greets her immediately, tail wagging with uncomplicated joy.

Nora kneels, letting the moment ground her.

Shoes off. Scrubs off.

She sits quietly, letting the day settle.

No monitors. No calculations.

Just stillness.

And the quiet understanding that today, precision protected the smallest patients.

Alignment Insight

Pediatric pharmacy is alignment through compassion and precision. Nora thrives in environments where careful attention and emotional presence intersect. Her alignment lives in protecting vulnerability with accuracy and care. Success is not measured in speed—it is measured in getting it exactly right.

24

#10 DAY IN THE LIFE — PSYCHIATRIC PHARMACIST

Name: Dr. Julian Mindwell, PharmD, BCPP — "The Quiet Stabilizer"

Scrub Color: Deep Indigo

Primary Role: Psychiatric Pharmacist (Inpatient Behavioral Health)

This Role Also Aligns With: Outpatient Mental Health Pharmacist (PharmD, BCPP); Addiction Medicine Pharmacist (PharmD, BCPP); Psychopharmacology Specialist (PharmD)

SCRUBfit™ Category: Med Heads

Pros: Deep patient impact; meaningful conversations; long-term stabilization; interdisciplinary respect.

Cons: Emotional complexity; slow progress; medication trial-and-error; stigma-related challenges.

Personality Traits: Patient, observant, empathetic, steady.

Clinical tools: Epic (gl); psychotropic medication guidelines; mood stabilization protocols; medication adherence tools; behavioral health documentation systems.

Clinical Confession: "In psychiatry, the smallest change in the right direction can be the biggest win."

Character Description

Dr. Julian Mindwell works in a space where progress is rarely immediate and often invisible. His Deep Indigo scrubs reflect the depth of the work—layered, complex, and not easily reduced to numbers or quick outcomes.

He understands that psychiatric pharmacy is not about fixing—it's about stabilizing, supporting, and guiding. Medications here are not just treatments; they are part of a broader process that includes trust, time, and careful adjustment.

Julian does not rush conversations. He listens longer than most. In a field where patients are often misunderstood or dismissed, that alone becomes part of the care.

Day in the Life (08:00–18:00)

06:20 — Wake-Up.

The alarm sounds softly, but Julian is already half-awake, drifting out of sleep gradually. The morning light is muted, the room quiet. He sits up slowly, taking a moment before moving.

At the foot of the bed, his gray tabby cat, Orion, stretches lazily, unconcerned with the start of the day. Julian smiles faintly. "You've got it figured out," he murmurs.

06:25 — First Moments.

He moves into the kitchen, starting coffee while the apartment remains still. No phone yet. No information overload. Just routine.

This is intentional. His work requires emotional presence, and that begins with protecting his own space first.

06:40 — Morning Routine.

He feeds Orion, watches him settle, and prepares a simple breakfast—toast, eggs, coffee. He eats slowly, seated, allowing himself to stay grounded before stepping into a world that often lacks stability.

06:55 — Mental Preparation.

He checks his schedule. Follow-up evaluations, medication adjustments, one new admission.

Psychiatric care doesn't move quickly—but it requires constant attention.

07:15 — Getting Ready.

Deep Indigo scrubs. Hair neat. Badge clipped. Minimal distraction.

He gathers his bag—tablet, notes, water bottle. Prepared, but not rushed.

07:30 — Commute.

The drive is calm, traffic steady but manageable. Julian listens to soft music, something consistent.

His mind shifts gradually—reviewing patient histories, medication responses, patterns of behavior.

This is not crisis management—it's continuity of care.

07:55 — Arrival.

He parks, sits for a brief moment, and takes a steady breath.

Then he steps inside.

08:00 — Unit Entry.

The behavioral health unit is quieter than most hospital floors, but the energy is different—less visible, more internal.

Julian logs into Epic (gl), reviewing overnight notes. Sleep patterns. Medication adherence. Behavioral observations.

These details matter here. They tell the real story.

08:30 — First Patient Review.

He meets with a patient adjusting to a new antidepressant.

"How have you been feeling?" he asks, voice calm, open.

The answer is not immediate. It rarely is.

He waits.

Eventually, the patient speaks.

That pause—that space—is part of the work.

10:00 — Medication Adjustment.

A patient experiencing side effects requires a dosing change.

Julian reviews the regimen carefully, considering both clinical data and patient experience.

He adjusts the dose—not drastically, but intentionally.

In psychiatry, small changes matter.

11:30 — Team Collaboration.

He meets with the care team—psychiatrists, nurses, social workers.

Discussion centers on progress, setbacks, next steps.

Julian contributes when needed, always measured, always clear.

12:45 — Lunch.

He eats quietly, not rushed, allowing himself a brief reset.

This pause is necessary. Emotional work requires recovery space.

13:30 — New Admission.

A new patient arrives, overwhelmed, uncertain.

Julian approaches carefully, introducing himself without urgency.

"We'll take this one step at a time," he says.

That reassurance is as important as any medication.

15:00 — Follow-Up Evaluations.

He meets with patients at different stages of progress. Some improving. Some plateauing. Some struggling.

Each interaction is different—but all require presence.

16:30 — Documentation.

He records notes carefully, capturing not just symptoms, but patterns and responses.

In this field, documentation supports continuity more than immediacy.

17:30 — End-of-Day Review.

He reviews medication plans, ensures clarity for the next shift, and prepares for handoff.

No loose ends.

18:00 — Badge Out.

He steps out into the evening air, the shift from internal intensity to external quiet immediate.

18:20 — Drive Home.

The car is quiet. Julian doesn't replay conversations—but certain moments stay with him.

A breakthrough. A hesitation. A small step forward.

18:40 — Home Reset.

Orion greets him at the door, weaving calmly between his legs.

Julian kneels, grounding himself in the moment.

Shoes off. Scrubs off.

He sits quietly, letting the day settle.

No expectations. No urgency.

Just stillness.

And the understanding that today, stability was built—one conversation at a time.

Alignment Insight

Psychiatric pharmacy is alignment through patience and presence. Julian thrives in environments where progress is measured in small, meaningful shifts. His alignment lives in listening, adjusting, and supporting over time. Success is not immediate—it is sustained.

25

#11 DAY IN THE LIFE — LONG-TERM CARE PHARMACIST

Name: Dr. Harold Carewell, PharmD, CGP — "The Continuity Guardian"

Scrub Color: Warm Sand

Primary Role: Long-Term Care Pharmacist (Skilled Nursing & Assisted Living Facilities)

This Role Also Aligns With: Consultant Pharmacist (PharmD, CGP); Geriatric Pharmacist (PharmD, CGP); Medication Therapy Management Specialist (PharmD)

SCRUBfit™ Category: Med Heads

Pros: Ongoing patient relationships; meaningful impact on quality of life; structured workflow; consultative role.

Cons: Polypharmacy complexity; slower system changes; regulatory requirements; limited immediate feedback.

Personality Traits: Patient, thorough, compassionate, detail-oriented.

Clinical tools: Electronic medication administration record (eMAR) (gl); consultant review platform; polypharmacy (gl) management tools; drug interaction databases; facility communication systems.

Clinical Confession: "In long-term care, safety isn't one decision

—it's hundreds of small ones made consistently."

Character Description

Dr. Harold Carewell moves through long-term care facilities with a quiet steadiness that reflects the pace of the environment itself. His Warm Sand scrubs blend into the calm, almost residential feel of the settings he visits—places where healthcare meets daily living.

He understands that his role is not about rapid intervention, but about sustained oversight. His patients are not passing through—they are staying, often for months or years. That changes everything.

For Harold, pharmacy is not about reacting to acute crises. It is about preventing slow-moving harm—subtle interactions, unnecessary medications, gradual declines that can be redirected with careful attention.

Day in the Life (08:00–17:30)

06:00 — Wake-Up.

Harold wakes to a soft alarm, the morning light already beginning to fill the room. He sits up slowly, giving himself a moment before standing. There is no rush in his mornings—he has learned that starting steady helps him stay steady.

At the foot of the bed, his aging golden retriever, Murphy, lifts his head slowly, tail wagging gently. Harold smiles. "Easy morning, my friend," he says quietly.

06:10 — First Routine.

He moves into the kitchen, starting coffee while Murphy follows closely behind. The house is quiet, the kind of quiet that feels settled rather than empty.

He fills Murphy's bowl, watching him eat at a slower pace than he once did. Time shows itself differently here—in small changes, subtle shifts.

06:25 — Breakfast.

Oatmeal, fruit, coffee. Harold eats at the table, reading through his notes for the day. Facility visits scheduled, medication reviews pending, regulatory checks required.

His work is structured—but never mechanical.

06:45 — Preparation.

He gathers his materials—tablet, printed reports, notes from previous reviews. Everything organized, everything accessible.

Long-term care requires continuity, and continuity requires preparation.

07:15 — Commute.

The drive is calm, roads lightly traveled. Harold listens to the radio at a low volume, more for background than engagement.

His mind moves through patient lists, recalling names, histories, medication patterns.

These are not new patients—they are ongoing stories.

07:50 — Arrival.

He parks outside the first facility, taking a brief moment before stepping out. No deep breath needed—just quiet readiness.

Then he walks in.

08:00 — Facility Entry.

The environment feels different from a hospital—less urgency, more routine. Staff greet him by name. Residents move through common areas slowly.

Harold logs into the eMAR (gl), pulling up medication profiles.

This is where his work begins—inside the details.

08:30 — Medication Review.

He scans through a resident's medication list. Multiple drugs. Overlapping indications. Potential interactions.

He pauses, focusing on one combination that doesn't sit right.

He reviews labs. Notes. Timing.

Then documents a recommendation: reduce dosage, monitor response.

Small adjustment. Long-term impact.

10:15 — Nurse Collaboration.

He meets with a nurse to discuss a resident's increasing confusion.

"Could be medication-related," Harold suggests gently.

They review the list together, identifying a possible contributor.

No immediate fix—but a clear direction.

11:30 — Resident Interaction.

He stops to speak with a resident he has seen for months.

"How are you feeling today?" he asks.

The conversation is simple—but meaningful.

In long-term care, presence matters.

12:30 — Lunch.

He eats in a quiet staff room, reviewing notes while he finishes his meal.

No rush—but no full disengagement either.

13:15 — Second Facility.

The afternoon brings a new location, new residents, but familiar patterns.

He logs in, begins again—reviewing, analyzing, adjusting.

Continuity extends across settings.

14:45 — Polypharmacy Review.

A complex case—multiple medications, overlapping effects.

Harold works through each one carefully, identifying what is necessary and what may no longer be.

Deprescribing is as important as prescribing here.

16:00 — Documentation and Recommendations.

He finalizes his notes, ensuring clarity for the care team.

What he writes must guide action—today, tomorrow, next week.

17:00 — Wrap-Up.

He reviews outstanding items, confirms follow-ups, prepares for the next visit.

No loose ends.

17:30 — End of Day.

He steps out of the facility into the quiet afternoon.

17:50 — Drive Home.

The road is steady, familiar. Harold reflects lightly—not on every detail, but on overall direction.

Are things improving? Stabilizing?

That's the measure here.

18:10 — Home Reset.

Murphy greets him slowly but warmly, tail wagging in quiet rhythm.

Harold kneels, grounding himself in the moment.

Shoes off. Work set aside.

He sits for a moment in stillness, letting the day settle naturally.

No urgency. No alarms.

Just continuity.

And the quiet understanding that today, steady care made a difference—one small adjustment at a time.

Alignment Insight

Long-term care pharmacy is alignment through consistency. Harold thrives in environments where patience and attention to detail shape outcomes over time. His alignment lives in continuity, prevention, and sustained care. Success is not immediate—it is gradual and lasting.

26

#12 DAY IN THE LIFE — SPECIALTY PHARMACY PHARMACIST

Name: Dr. Aria Scriptwell, PharmD — "The Access Navigator"

Scrub Color: Sapphire Stream

Primary Role: Specialty Pharmacy Pharmacist (High-Cost / Complex Therapies)

This Role Also Aligns With: Clinical Pharmacist (PharmD); Patient Access Pharmacist (PharmD); Prior Authorization Specialist (PharmD)

SCRUBfit™ Category: Med Heads

Pros: High-impact therapies; patient advocacy; measurable outcomes; coordinated care.

Cons: Insurance complexity; administrative burden; access delays; emotional frustration.

Personality Traits: Persistent, detail-driven, empathetic, solution-oriented.

Clinical tools: Specialty pharmacy management platform; prior authorization (gl) systems; benefits investigation tools; patient assistance program databases; Epic (gl); payer portals.

Clinical Confession: "Sometimes the hardest part isn't the medication—it's getting the patient to it."

Character Description

Dr. Aria Scriptwell operates in a space where medicine meets access, and access is never guaranteed. Her Sapphire Stream scrubs reflect the constant movement required in her role—flowing between systems, providers, insurers, and patients.

She knows that the most advanced therapies in the world mean nothing if patients cannot receive them. That reality shapes everything she does.

For Aria, pharmacy is not just clinical—it is navigational. Every approval, every appeal, every resolved barrier becomes part of the treatment itself.

Day in the Life (08:30–18:00)

06:25 — Wake-Up.

Aria's alarm sounds softly, but she reaches for it immediately. The room is still, early light just beginning to filter in. She sits up slowly, taking a moment before the day begins.

At the edge of the bed, her orange tabby, Sol, stretches lazily, completely unconcerned with urgency. Aria smiles faintly. "You've got the easier job," she says quietly.

06:30 — Morning Routine.

She moves into the kitchen, starting coffee while the apartment remains calm. This quiet is intentional—her work will not be.

She feeds Sol, watches him settle, then prepares a simple breakfast—toast, eggs, coffee. She eats sitting down, grounding herself before stepping into complexity.

06:50 — First Check-In.

She opens her tablet, reviewing pending cases.

Denied authorization.

Pending appeal.

Urgent therapy request.

Her expression sharpens—not frustrated, but focused.

This is where her day begins.

07:10 — Getting Ready.

Sapphire Stream scrubs. Hair secured. Badge clipped.

She checks her bag—tablet, notes, backup pen. Everything she needs to navigate the system ahead.

07:30 — Commute.

Traffic builds steadily, but Aria remains composed. She listens to light music, letting her mind transition gradually.

She reviews cases mentally—not clinical dosing, but access pathways.

Who needs escalation?

What requires follow-up?

This is strategy, not just medicine.

08:25 — Arrival Pause.

She sits briefly in the car, reviewing her top priority cases.

One patient stands out—urgent therapy delayed by insurance denial.

She exhales once.

Then steps in.

08:30 — System Entry.

She logs into the specialty pharmacy platform, pulling up active cases.

Each case is layered—clinical need, insurance requirements, administrative steps.

Her role is to connect them all.

09:00 — Prior Authorization Push.

She begins with the most urgent case.

Reviewing documentation. Matching criteria. Submitting additional clinical justification.

Every word matters. Every detail must align.

This is not just paperwork—it's access.

10:30 — Provider Coordination.

She calls a physician's office to clarify documentation.

"Can you update the note to reflect failed therapies?" she asks.

Without that detail, approval won't happen.

Small change. Major impact.

11:45 — Patient Call.

She speaks with a patient waiting for approval.

"I know it's frustrating," she says calmly. "We're pushing this forward."

Reassurance is part of the job.

The delay is not her fault—but she carries it with the patient anyway.

12:45 — Lunch.

She eats quickly, reviewing notes between bites.

No full pause—just a brief reset.

13:30 — Appeal Submission.

A denied case requires escalation.

She builds the appeal carefully—clinical data, prior failures, justification.

This is where persistence matters most.

15:00 — Breakthrough Moment.

An approval comes through.

She pauses for just a second, allowing herself to register it.

Then moves immediately—coordinating delivery, notifying the patient.

This is the reward.

16:30 — Follow-Up Loop.

She checks remaining cases, ensuring nothing stalls.

Momentum must be maintained.

17:30 — Final Review.

She updates documentation, confirms next steps, prepares for the following day.

No loose ends.

18:00 — Badge Out.

She steps out into the evening air, the mental intensity fading gradually.

18:20 — Drive Home.

The car is quiet. Aria lets the day settle—not replaying everything, but acknowledging what moved forward.

18:40 — Home Reset.

Sol greets her instantly, weaving between her legs.

She kneels, grounding herself in the moment.

Shoes off. Work aside.

She sits quietly, letting the stillness return.

No systems. No barriers.

Just calm.

And the understanding that today, persistence turned possibility into access.

Alignment Insight

Specialty pharmacy is alignment through advocacy. Aria thrives in navigating complexity and removing barriers to care. Her alignment lives in persistence, strategy, and patient support. Success is not just clinical—it is making treatment possible.

27

#13 DAY IN THE LIFE — NUCLEAR PHARMACIST

Name: Dr. Victor Halfman, PharmD, BCNP — "The Precision Isotope"

Scrub Color: Graphite Silver

Primary Role: Nuclear Pharmacist (Radiopharmaceutical Compounding & Distribution)

This Role Also Aligns With: Radiopharmacy Specialist (PharmD, BCNP); PET Imaging Pharmacist (PharmD); Quality & Safety Lead (Radiopharmacy)

SCRUBfit™ Category: Med Heads

Pros: Highly specialized practice; predictable workflow; strong quality controls; critical role in diagnostic imaging.

Cons: Early hours; strict regulatory environment; radiation safety requirements; limited patient interaction.

Personality Traits: Meticulous, disciplined, process-oriented, calm.

Clinical tools: Dose calibrator (gl); laminar airflow hood; hot cell (gl); Geiger counter (gl); lead shielding; radiopharmaceutical kits; transport containers; time-activity charts.

Clinical Confession: "In nuclear pharmacy, timing isn't important —it's everything."

Character Description

Dr. Victor Halfman operates in a world where precision is measured in seconds and decay is a constant reality. His Graphite Silver scrubs reflect the controlled, highly regulated environment he works within—one where every movement is deliberate and every process is exact.

Unlike most pharmacy roles, his work begins before the rest of the healthcare system fully wakes. By the time imaging departments open, his work must already be complete, verified, and delivered.

For Victor, pharmacy is not about reacting—it is about executing flawlessly within constraints that cannot be adjusted. Time moves in one direction here, and there are no second chances.

Day in the Life (03:30–13:30)

02:45 — Wake-Up.

The alarm sounds in the dark, long before sunrise. Victor reaches for it immediately, silencing it before it can echo.

There is no hesitation. This schedule is not negotiable—it is part of the role.

The room is silent, the world outside still asleep.

02:50 — First Movement.

He sits up, fully awake within seconds. Routine has trained his body to adapt.

In the corner, his sleek black cat, Onyx, watches quietly, accustomed to these early starts.

Victor nods slightly, acknowledging the presence without breaking rhythm.

02:55 — Morning Routine.

He moves through the kitchen with minimal light, starting coffee and preparing a simple breakfast.

No distractions. No unnecessary steps.

Everything is efficient, intentional.

03:05 — Mental Preparation.

He reviews the day's schedule on his tablet.

Radiopharmaceutical orders. Delivery timelines. Decay curves.

Every dose must be prepared within a precise window.

There is no flexibility—only accuracy.

03:15 — Getting Ready.

Graphite Silver scrubs. Badge secured. Radiation monitoring badge clipped carefully into place.

He checks his bag—notes, identification, essentials.

Preparation is part of safety.

03:20 — Commute.

The roads are empty, the city silent.

Victor drives without music, his mind already aligned with the day's demands.

Timing. Sequence. Precision.

03:30 — Arrival.

He parks outside the radiopharmacy, the building quiet and controlled.

No pause needed. He steps directly into motion.

03:30 — Entry and Setup.

Inside, the environment is sterile, regulated, exact.

Victor logs in, checks radiation levels, verifies equipment readiness.

Every step follows protocol.

03:45 — Dose Preparation Begins.

He begins compounding radiopharmaceuticals, working within the hot cell (gl), shielded and controlled.

Movements are deliberate—no wasted motion, no deviation.

Time is already a factor. Decay has started.

05:00 — Calibration Check.

Each dose is measured using the dose calibrator (gl), ensuring precise activity levels.

Too high—adjust.

Too low—recalculate.

There is no approximation.

06:15 — Quality Assurance.

He verifies each preparation, documenting meticulously.

Accuracy is not assumed—it is proven.

07:00 — Distribution Coordination.

Transport containers are prepared, shielded, labeled, and scheduled.

Delivery timing must align perfectly with imaging appointments.

A delay here affects everything downstream.

08:30 — Final Batch Completion.

The last doses are prepared, verified, and released.

Victor reviews all documentation once more, ensuring nothing has been missed.

09:15 — Facility Check.

He monitors radiation levels, ensuring safety standards remain intact.

Every environment must remain controlled.

10:30 — Documentation Block.

He completes detailed records of all preparations, calibrations, and distributions.

This documentation is as critical as the work itself.

11:45 — Equipment Maintenance.

He performs routine checks on equipment, ensuring readiness for the next cycle.

Consistency depends on reliability.

12:30 — Wrap-Up.

He reviews the day's work, confirming all processes were completed correctly.

No loose ends.

13:30 — End of Shift.

Victor removes his radiation badge, secures equipment, and exits the facility.

13:50 — Drive Home.

The world is fully awake now—traffic, movement, noise.

Victor drives through it quietly, already transitioning out of precision mode.

14:10 — Home Reset.

Onyx greets him silently, weaving through his legs.

Victor sets his bag down, removes his shoes, and sits for a moment.

No alarms. No timers. No decay curves.

Just stillness.

And the quiet understanding that today, precision held firm—exactly as it needed to.

Alignment Insight

Nuclear pharmacy is alignment through precision and discipline. Victor thrives in environments where timing, control, and exact execution define success. His alignment lives in process, accuracy, and consistency. Success is not visible—it is exact.

28

#14 DAY IN THE LIFE — PHARMACOVIGILANCE PHARMACIST

Name: Dr. Elena Safeguard, PharmD, MS — "The Signal Watcher"

Scrub Color: Midnight Violet

Primary Role: Pharmacovigilance Pharmacist (Drug Safety & Adverse Event Monitoring)

This Role Also Aligns With: Drug Safety Specialist (PharmD); Regulatory Affairs Pharmacist (PharmD, MS); Clinical Data Analyst (PharmD, MPH)

SCRUBfit™ Category: Med Heads

Pros: System-wide patient safety impact; analytical work; structured environment; influence on policy and labeling.

Cons: Indirect patient contact; data-heavy workload; delayed feedback loops; regulatory complexity.

Personality Traits: Analytical, observant, detail-oriented, quietly persistent.

Clinical tools: Safety databases; adverse event reporting systems; signal detection software; regulatory reporting platforms; data visualization tools; literature review databases.

Clinical Confession: "Most people never see what I do—but when something goes wrong, it's already too late to start looking."

Character Description

Dr. Elena Safeguard works in a space where the patient is not in front of her—but is always present in the data she reviews. Her Midnight Violet scrubs reflect the depth of her work—quiet, layered, and often unseen.

She understands that drug safety is not reactive—it is anticipatory. Every report she reviews, every signal she evaluates, contributes to a broader understanding of how medications behave outside controlled environments.

For Elena, pharmacy is about patterns—detecting subtle shifts before they become widespread harm. Her work is not dramatic, but it is essential.

Day in the Life (08:30–17:30)

06:40 — Wake-Up.

Elena wakes to a soft alarm, the room filled with early morning light. She lies still for a moment, allowing her mind to come online gradually.

At the edge of the bed, her Siamese cat, Lyra, stretches elegantly, already alert. Elena smiles faintly. "You're ahead of me," she says quietly.

06:45 — Morning Routine.

She moves into the kitchen, starting coffee while the apartment remains calm. No immediate phone check. No rush into data.

This quiet is intentional—her work requires sustained focus, and that begins with a clear mind.

07:00 — Breakfast.

She prepares a simple meal—fruit, yogurt, coffee—and sits at the table to eat. No multitasking. No screens.

This is her baseline—calm before analysis.

07:20 — First Data Check.

She opens her tablet, reviewing overnight safety alerts.

Adverse event reports. Signal flags. Literature updates.

Her expression sharpens slightly—not reactive, but attentive.

Patterns don't announce themselves—they must be noticed.

07:45 — Getting Ready.

Midnight Violet scrubs. Hair secured. Badge clipped.

She gathers her materials—tablet, notes, reference documents.

Preparation is mental as much as physical.

08:05 — Commute.

Traffic is steady, predictable. Elena listens to instrumental music, something that supports focus without distraction.

Her mind begins to organize the day's priorities—signal review, case evaluation, reporting deadlines.

08:25 — Arrival Pause.

She sits briefly in the car, reviewing top alerts.

One cluster stands out—similar adverse reactions across multiple reports.

She exhales once.

Then steps in.

08:30 — System Entry.

She logs into the safety database, pulling up new case reports.

Each report represents a real patient experience—symptoms, outcomes, timelines.

Her job is to connect them.

09:15 — Case Review.

She reads through detailed reports, noting patterns—timing of onset, severity, co-medications.

Nothing is dismissed. Every detail matters.

10:45 — Signal Detection.

Using specialized software, she evaluates trends across multiple cases.

A possible signal begins to emerge—subtle, but consistent.

She leans forward slightly, focus sharpening.

This is where her work matters most.

12:15 — Lunch.

She eats quietly, reviewing notes. No full disengagement—just a brief pause in intensity.

13:00 — Team Collaboration.

She meets with a small team to discuss emerging signals.

"Elena, what are you seeing?" a colleague asks.

She presents clearly—data, patterns, interpretation.

Discussion follows, measured and analytical.

14:30 — Regulatory Reporting.

She prepares documentation for reporting requirements, ensuring accuracy and completeness.

What she writes may influence labeling, warnings, future use.

Precision matters.

15:45 — Literature Review.

She scans recent publications, comparing findings with observed data.

External evidence strengthens internal observations.

16:45 — Final Review.

She revisits key cases, confirming conclusions and next steps.

No assumptions. Only verified patterns.

17:30 — End of Day.

She logs out, closing the system with a sense of completion—not finality, but progression.

17:50 — Drive Home.

The car is quiet. Elena reflects lightly—not on individual cases, but on patterns emerging.

18:10 — Home Reset.

Lyra greets her calmly, weaving around her legs.

Elena kneels briefly, grounding herself in the moment.

Shoes off. Work set aside.

She sits quietly, letting the day settle.

No data streams. No alerts.

Just stillness.

And the quiet understanding that today, unseen patterns moved closer to clarity.

Alignment Insight

Pharmacovigilance is alignment through awareness. Elena thrives in environments where analysis and pattern recognition drive patient safety. Her alignment lives in detail, persistence, and quiet impact. Success is not immediate—it is preventive.

29

#15 DAY IN THE LIFE — PHARMACEUTICAL INDUSTRY PHARMACIST

Name: Dr. Sebastian Vantrell, PharmD, MBA — "The Pipeline Architect"

Scrub Color: Obsidian Black

Primary Role: Pharmaceutical Industry Pharmacist (Medical Affairs / Clinical Strategy)

This Role Also Aligns With: Medical Science Liaison (PharmD); Clinical Development Pharmacist (PharmD, PhD); Regulatory Strategy Lead (PharmD, MBA)

SCRUBfit™ Category: Med Heads

Pros: Broad impact across populations; strategic influence; higher earning potential; structured schedule.

Cons: Indirect patient contact; corporate pressure; travel demands; performance expectations.

Personality Traits: Strategic, articulate, analytical, relationship-driven.

Clinical tools: Clinical trial data platforms; CRM systems; literature databases; presentation software; regulatory documentation systems; virtual meeting platforms.

Clinical Confession: "You don't treat one patient—you shape how thousands will be treated."

Character Description

Dr. Sebastian Vantrell operates in a world far removed from bedside care, yet deeply connected to it. His Obsidian Black scrubs are more symbolic than functional—reflecting the polished, structured environment of the pharmaceutical industry.

He understands that his decisions do not play out in a single room, but across entire systems—clinical trials, treatment protocols, provider education. His work influences how therapies are understood, adopted, and ultimately used.

For Sebastian, pharmacy is no longer about individual interventions. It is about shaping the trajectory of medicine itself.

Day in the Life (07:30–18:30)

05:45 — Wake-Up.

Sebastian's alarm sounds clean and precise, matching the structure of his day ahead. He silences it immediately, sitting up without hesitation.

The room is quiet, city light filtering through the window. He takes a moment—not to linger, but to orient.

At the foot of the bed, his sleek Siamese cat, Vale, stretches slowly, watching him with calm interest.

"Early start," Sebastian says quietly, already moving.

05:50 — Morning Routine.

He moves into the kitchen, starting espresso with practiced efficiency. Everything about his routine is intentional—measured, controlled.

Breakfast is simple but deliberate—protein, fruit, coffee. He eats seated, reviewing his calendar for the day.

Meetings. Data review. Strategy calls.

No surprises—but plenty of pressure.

06:10 — First Review.

He opens his tablet, scanning overnight updates from global teams.

Clinical trial data. Market feedback. Regulatory notes.

His expression sharpens slightly.

This is where his day begins—not with patients, but with information.

06:30 — Getting Ready.

Obsidian Black scrubs—symbolic of his clinical roots—paired with a structured jacket. Badge clipped. Watch set.

He gathers his materials—laptop, notes, presentation files.

Preparation here is strategic, not procedural.

06:50 — Commute.

The city is already moving. Traffic builds, but Sebastian remains composed.

He listens to a recorded briefing, absorbing updates while driving.

His mind shifts into strategy mode—connecting data points, anticipating questions.

07:25 — Arrival Pause.

He sits briefly in the car, reviewing his top priorities.

One key meeting stands out—data presentation to senior leadership.

He exhales once.

Then steps out.

07:30 — Office Entry.

The environment is controlled, polished, structured.

Sebastian logs in, pulling up clinical data dashboards.

Everything is organized—but the stakes are high.

08:00 — Data Review.

He analyzes trial results, focusing on efficacy, safety, and trends.

Numbers tell a story—but interpretation shapes the outcome.

He leans forward slightly, refining his understanding.

09:30 — Strategy Meeting.

He joins a virtual call with cross-functional teams.

"Based on the data, we may need to adjust positioning," he says clearly.

Discussion follows—measured, strategic, deliberate.

11:00 — Medical Affairs Call.

He speaks with external providers, discussing clinical findings and implications.

Clarity is critical—how information is communicated affects adoption.

12:30 — Lunch.

He eats at his desk, reviewing notes between bites.

No full pause—just continuation.

13:15 — Presentation Preparation.

He refines slides for an upcoming leadership meeting.

Every detail matters—data accuracy, wording, visual clarity.

This is where strategy becomes communication.

15:00 — Leadership Presentation.

He presents findings to senior leadership.

Confident. Structured. Precise.

Questions come quickly.

He responds without hesitation, grounded in data.

16:30 — Follow-Up Actions.

He reviews feedback, adjusts plans, coordinates next steps.

Momentum must be maintained.

17:30 — Final Review.

He checks outstanding items, ensuring alignment across teams.

No loose ends.

18:30 — End of Day.

He logs out, closing the laptop with a sense of controlled completion.

18:50 — Drive Home.

The city is still active, but his pace slows.

He reflects lightly—not on individuals, but on impact.

19:10 — Home Reset.

Vale greets him quietly, weaving through his legs.

Sebastian sets his bag down, removes his jacket, and sits for a moment.

No meetings. No data. No expectations.

Just stillness.

And the understanding that today, strategy shaped the direction of care—far beyond a single patient.

Alignment Insight

Pharmaceutical industry pharmacy is alignment through strategy and scale. Sebastian thrives in environments where data, communication, and influence shape outcomes across populations. His alignment lives in big-picture thinking and execution. Success is not immediate—it is far-reaching.

30

PREREQUISITES TO BECOMING A PHARMACIST

Prerequisites to Becoming a Pharmacist

If you are drawn to both the science of medications and the real-world impact those medications have on patients, pharmacy offers a path where chemistry, clinical reasoning, and patient counseling all collide. In the United States, "pharmacist" is a tightly regulated professional title. To earn it, you follow a pathway that moves from pre-pharmacy coursework to a Doctor of Pharmacy (PharmD) degree, then on to national board exams and state licensure. Each step is designed to prove that you can safely manage powerful therapies and guide patients through using them.

The journey typically begins with pre-pharmacy study at a college or university. Some students complete a full bachelor's degree before entering pharmacy school, while others follow a two- or three-year pre-pharmacy track that satisfies the required prerequisites. Either way, the early years are heavy on science and math. You can expect multiple semesters of general and organic chemistry with labs, general biology, human anatomy and physiology, microbiology, calculus, and statistics. Many schools also require or strongly recommend physics, biochemistry, economics, public speaking, and written communication. These courses do more than check boxes; they give you the scientific vocabulary and quantitative habits you will rely on when you are adjusting doses, interpreting lab results, and catching potentially dangerous drug interactions.

Academic performance in this phase matters. Pharmacy programs typically set minimum GPA standards and look closely at how you performed in your science and math courses. A rough semester is not an automatic barrier, but the PharmD curriculum is dense and fast-moving. Admissions committees want to see that you can handle complex material, stay organized, and recover from setbacks. An upward trend in grades, strong results in upper-division courses, and thoughtful letters of recommendation all help tell that story.

Once your foundational coursework is in place, the key prerequisite becomes admission to an accredited Doctor of Pharmacy program. PharmD programs in the United States are generally four years long and are accredited by the Accreditation Council for Pharmacy Education. Admission decisions are based on your college transcript, prerequisite completion, personal statement, references, and a detailed record of your experiences. Some programs once required a standardized test such as the PCAT, but many have moved away from that requirement and now place more emphasis on holistic review and evidence of readiness for a professional health program.

Experiences outside the classroom are powerful prerequisites in their own right. Working or volunteering in pharmacy settings—as a pharmacy technician, pharmacy assistant, or volunteer—helps you understand the day-to-day reality behind the counter and in the hospital med room. You see how prescriptions flow through the system, how pharmacists collaborate with physicians and nurses, and how counseling conversations actually unfold at the window. Experience in other healthcare roles, such as patient care technician, medical assistant, or community health worker, can also strengthen an application by showing that you are comfortable around patients, understand professional boundaries, and can communicate clearly in stressful situations.

Inside the PharmD program, your focus shifts from getting in to proving your competence. The curriculum blends classroom learning with extensive experiential education. You study pharmacology, pharmaceutics, medicinal chemistry, pharmacotherapy across body systems, pathophysiology, law and ethics, public health, communication skills, and pharmacy management. At the same time, you complete structured clinical rotations in settings like hospitals, community pharmacies, ambulatory care clinics, long-term care facilities, and sometimes industry or research environments. These advanced practice experiences are where you learn to apply your knowledge: reviewing medication profiles, checking for interactions, making dosing recommendations, counseling patients, and collaborating with interprofessional care teams.

By the time you approach graduation, the last set of prerequisites is tied to licensure. Every aspiring pharmacist must pass a national licensure examination that tests general pharmacy practice knowledge, and in most states, a separate law exam that covers federal and state pharmacy regulations. States also require completion of a set number of supervised internship or practice hours, some of which are built into the PharmD program and some of which are tracked separately through boards of pharmacy. In addition, many states require background checks and documentation of your education and good standing.

When you put it all together, the prerequisites to becoming a pharmacist form a long but coherent arc. You build a rigorous science and math foundation, demonstrate academic reliability, gain first-hand experience in pharmacy and healthcare settings, complete a professional doctoral program, and then prove your readiness through national and state licensing requirements. The purpose is not to make the path difficult for its own sake, but to ensure that when a patient hands you a prescription—or asks if two medications are safe to take together—you have the depth of training, judgment, and confidence to answer well.

31

WHAT I WISH I HAD KNOWN

What I Wish I Had Known When I Started as a Pharmacist

When I first became a Pharmacist, I thought my role was to count pills and verify orders. I believed success would come down to memorization, speed, and accuracy alone. And while those things matter, they are only the surface of what this profession truly demands. I quickly learned that pharmacy is far more than math and medicine — it's the science of safety, the language of trust, and the art of stewardship. Every dose you approve or question carries weight, even when the moment feels routine. What seems like a small decision in your workflow can become a defining moment in someone else's life. You begin to understand that you are not just processing medications — you are shaping outcomes, often in ways you will never directly witness.

I wish I had known that accuracy is compassion in disguise. In school, accuracy feels technical — numbers, formulas, correct answers. In practice, it becomes deeply human. Behind every decimal point, every recalculation, every moment you pause instead of rushing forward is a patient depending on you to get it right. The work is quiet, often unnoticed, but it is never insignificant. You may never meet the person whose outcome changed because of something you caught, something you questioned, or something you refused to ignore. But that doesn't make it invisible — it makes it foundational. Accuracy is not just precision; it is protection. It is one of the purest forms of care you will ever deliver.

I wish someone had told me that you'll be both invisible and indispensable at the same time. There will be days when your work feels like it exists in the background — behind screens, within systems, inside workflows that move quickly past your contributions. People may see the medication, but not the thinking behind it. They may see the order completed, but not the risk that was prevented. And yet, within that invisibility, you will become essential. The system depends on you to notice what others cannot, to question what others may accept, and to hold a standard that does not bend under pressure. You will learn to find pride not in recognition, but in reliability. Not in being seen, but in being trusted.

I wish I had realized sooner that collaboration is as vital as calculation. Pharmacy is not a siloed profession, even if parts of the work feel independent. The strongest pharmacists are not just accurate — they are communicators, educators, and partners in care. You will speak with nurses who are managing complex patients, physicians who are balancing multiple priorities, and colleagues who rely on your expertise to guide decisions. Over time, you will learn that how you say something matters just as much as what you say. Your knowledge becomes more powerful when it is shared effectively. Collaboration transforms information into action, and action into outcomes.

I wish I had known that the pressure never fully goes away — and that's not something to fear. Early on, that pressure can feel overwhelming. The responsibility, the constant need for accuracy, the awareness that mistakes matter — it can feel heavy. But over time, you begin to understand that this pressure is not a weakness. It is a signal that you care. It is the internal standard that keeps you sharp, focused, and accountable. The goal is not to eliminate pressure, but to work within it. To channel it into preparation, into discipline, into consistency. Pharmacy is not about being comfortable — it is about being dependable, even when the stakes are high.

I wish someone had told me how much your empathy would be tested. Not just by patients, but by systems. By medication shortages that limit options. By policies that complicate care. By long hours where the workload never fully lets up. You will feel the tension between doing what is ideal and what is possible. And in those moments, you will learn that perfection is not the goal — intention is. You do the best you can with the information, resources, and time you have. You advocate when you can, adjust when you must, and stay grounded in the purpose behind the work. Empathy in pharmacy is not just emotional — it is practical, steady, and resilient.

I wish I had understood earlier how much growth in this profession comes from experience, not just knowledge. There is a difference between knowing something and recognizing it in real time. At first, everything feels deliberate — every decision requires effort, every scenario feels new. But over time, patterns begin to emerge. You notice trends faster. You recognize risks sooner. You respond with greater clarity. Confidence builds, not because the work becomes easier, but because you become more capable within it. That growth is gradual, but it is real. And it is one of the most rewarding parts of the journey.

I wish I had known that not every day will feel meaningful in the moment. Some days will feel routine. Repetitive. Heavy with small tasks that don't seem significant on their own. But meaning in pharmacy is cumulative. It builds over time, through consistency, through reliability, through the quiet prevention of harm. You don't measure your impact in single moments — you measure it in patterns. In the absence of errors. In the stability of patients. In the trust of your team. Over time, those small, steady contributions become something much larger.

And most of all, I wish I had known that being a Pharmacist is one of the most quietly heroic roles in healthcare. You are the guardian of safety in a system that depends on precision. You are the translator of complexity in a field that often overwhelms. You are the calm voice in moments where clarity matters most. One day, someone will say, "Good catch," or "Thank you for that," and it may seem small. But in that moment, you will understand the weight of what you do. You may not always be seen, but you are always essential.

Because at its heart, pharmacy isn't about dispensing drugs — it's about dispensing trust, precision, and hope. And once you understand that, the work changes. Not in what you do, but in how deeply you understand why it matters.

32

ALIGNMENT AND AVOIDING BURNOUT

Staying in the Role Without Losing Yourself

One of the most important things I wish I had understood earlier in my career is this: burnout is not always about working too hard — it is often about working in a way that does not fit who you are.

Pharmacy is a demanding profession. The pace can be intense, the expectations are high, and the margin for error is small. But not every pharmacist experiences that pressure the same way. Some thrive in fast-paced, high-acuity environments. Others find their rhythm in structured, predictable settings. The difference is not capability — it is alignment.

When your role matches how you are wired, the work feels sustainable. When it doesn't, even a "good job" can become exhausting over time.

Understanding that distinction changes everything.

Burnout Doesn't Start Where You Think It Does

Most people assume burnout begins with long hours or heavy workloads. Those factors matter, but they are not the root cause. Burnout often starts much earlier — in the quiet friction between what the job demands and what you naturally need to function well.

You might feel it as:

- Constant mental fatigue, even on lighter days
- Irritation that doesn't seem proportional to the situation
- A sense of being "on" all the time, with no real reset
- Loss of satisfaction in work that once felt meaningful

These are not signs that you are failing. They are signals that something is misaligned.

Ignoring those signals does not make them go away — it amplifies them.

The Role Matters Less Than the Fit

One of the most common mistakes in pharmacy is choosing a role based on external factors alone — salary, prestige, or perceived opportunity — without considering daily experience.

Two pharmacists can have the same title and completely different lives.

One may feel energized, engaged, and challenged in a positive way.

The other may feel drained, overwhelmed, and disconnected.

The difference is not the job. It is the fit between the person and the environment.

Some pharmacists are wired for:

- Fast-paced, high-pressure environments (Emergency, ICU)
- Deep, analytical work (Infectious Disease, Pharmacovigilance)
- Long-term patient relationships (Ambulatory Care, Long-Term Care)
- Structured, system-based roles (Industry, Specialty Pharmacy)

There is no "best" path — only the path that fits you best.

Know How You Work — Not Just What You Know

Pharmacy education teaches you what to know. Experience teaches you how to work. Alignment comes from understanding both.

Ask yourself:

- Do I prefer urgency or predictability?
- Do I thrive on constant interaction or focused independent work?

- Do I want immediate impact or long-term influence?
- How much pressure feels energizing vs. overwhelming?

These questions are not abstract — they define whether your career will feel sustainable.

Ignoring them leads to misalignment.

Understanding them creates direction.

Energy Is a Better Metric Than Hours

Instead of asking, "How many hours am I working?" ask, "What is this work taking out of me?"

Two roles can have the same schedule but completely different energy demands.

One may leave you mentally drained.

Another may leave you focused but satisfied.

Energy is shaped by:

- Cognitive load (constant decision-making vs. structured tasks)
- Emotional load (patient interaction, difficult conversations)
- Environmental stress (interruptions, pace, expectations)

Managing burnout requires managing energy, not just time.

Small Adjustments Matter More Than Big Changes

Not every solution requires leaving your role. Sometimes, small adjustments create meaningful improvement.

This might look like:

- Shifting responsibilities within your current position
- Adjusting your workflow to reduce unnecessary friction
- Setting clearer boundaries around availability
- Developing more efficient systems for repetitive tasks

These changes may seem minor, but they compound over time.

Burnout often develops gradually — and it can be reduced the same way.

Boundaries Are a Professional Skill

In pharmacy, there is always more to do. More orders to review. More questions to answer. More problems to solve.

Without boundaries, the work expands indefinitely.

Setting boundaries does not mean doing less — it means protecting your ability to do your work well.

This includes:

- Taking breaks when possible
- Avoiding unnecessary overextension
- Recognizing when your capacity is reached

Sustainable performance depends on knowing your limits — and respecting them.

You Are Not Supposed to Be Perfect

Perfectionism is common in pharmacy, but it is not sustainable.

You are expected to be accurate, thorough, and responsible — not flawless.

There will be moments where:

- Information is incomplete
- Decisions are complex
- Outcomes are uncertain

In those moments, the goal is not perfection — it is sound judgment.

Letting go of perfectionism reduces unnecessary pressure while maintaining high standards.

Support Systems Are Not Optional

Pharmacy can feel isolating, especially in high-responsibility roles. Having a support system — both inside and outside of work — is essential.

This includes:

- Colleagues who understand the work
- Mentors who provide guidance
- Personal connections that allow you to disconnect

No one sustains this profession alone.

Connection is part of resilience.

Recognizing When It's Time to Pivot

Sometimes, burnout is not something to fix — it is something to listen to.

If you consistently feel:

- Drained regardless of workload
- Disconnected from the purpose of your work
- Unable to recover between shifts

It may not be a matter of adjustment. It may be a matter of direction.

Pharmacy offers multiple pathways. Moving to a different setting is not failure — it is alignment.

The goal is not to endure the wrong fit.

It is to find the right one.

Bringing It Back to Alignment

This is where alignment becomes more than an idea — it becomes a practical framework for decision-making.

When evaluating your role, ask:

- Does this environment match how I function best?
- Is the pace sustainable for me long-term?
- Does the type of work align with what gives me energy?

If the answer is consistently no, the issue is not your ability.

It is the mismatch between the role and your design.

And that can be changed.

The Long View

A career in pharmacy is not defined by a single role. It is a series of decisions, adjustments, and transitions over time.

You will evolve.

Your preferences will change.

Your definition of success will shift.

What matters is not finding the perfect role immediately.

It is staying aware enough to adjust when something no longer fits.

Burnout is not a sign that you are not capable.

It is a signal that something needs to change.

And when you respond to that signal — thoughtfully, intentionally — you move closer to a career that is not just successful, but sustainable.

33

BEFORE YOU APPLY TO PHARMACY SCHOOL™

What People Wish They Had Known

Choosing to become a pharmacist is not just an academic decision.

It is a financial decision.

A lifestyle decision.

An identity decision.

And for many people, the most important parts of that decision are not fully understood until after they have already committed.

This chapter exists to change that.

Not to discourage you.

Not to persuade you.

But to give you a clearer, more complete picture—before you invest years of your life and significant financial resources into this path.

A Pharmacist Reflects

When I first became a Pharmacist, I thought my role was to count pills and verify orders. I quickly learned that pharmacy is far more than math and medicine — it's the science of safety, the language of trust, and the art of stewardship. Every dose you approve or question ripples through someone's life in ways you may never see.

I wish I had known that accuracy is compassion in disguise. Behind every decimal, every double-check, every intercepted error is a patient who may never know how close they came to harm. Your vigilance isn't invisible — it's lifesaving. You may not be at the bedside, but you're always part of the heartbeat.

I wish someone had told me that you'll be both invisible and indispensable. People often see the pills, not the person behind the verification queue, the drug interaction caught at 2 a.m., or the policy you rewrote after a near miss. But the quiet work of pharmacy is often the difference between good care and great care. You are the unseen advocate in the medication story.

I wish I'd realized sooner that collaboration is as vital as calculation. The best pharmacists don't work in silos; they round, they explain, they teach, they listen. You'll learn that your credibility doesn't come from how much you know, but from how well you communicate it. Every nurse who calls you, every physician who seeks your input, is a reminder that your knowledge builds bridges, not barriers.

I wish I had known that the pressure never fully goes away — and that's okay. The weight you feel before approving a chemo regimen or a pediatric dose isn't fear; it's integrity. It means you care. Channel that tension into thoroughness, not self-doubt. Pharmacy is precision under pressure, purpose under protocol.

I wish someone had told me that your empathy will be tested — by shortages, by policies, by long hours, by the constant pull between doing more and doing right. You'll find peace not in perfection, but in knowing that every decision you make is guided by care, evidence, and conscience.

And most of all, I wish I had known that being a Pharmacist is one of the most quietly heroic roles in healthcare. You'll be the guardian of safety, the translator of complexity, and the calm voice in moments of uncertainty. One day, when a provider says, "Good catch," or a patient's pain is finally controlled because you insisted on the right regimen, you'll realize something powerful: you may not always be seen, but you are always essential.

Because at its heart, pharmacy isn't about dispensing drugs — it's about dispensing trust, precision, and hope.

THE FINANCIAL COMMITMENT **Is Real**

Before you ever step into a pharmacy, you will make one of the largest financial decisions of your life.

A Doctor of Pharmacy (PharmD) degree often comes with:

- Six to eight years of education
- Tuition that can exceed $150,000–$250,000
- Additional living expenses and lost earning years

This is not just a number on paper.

It becomes part of your life:

- It influences where you work
- It affects how quickly you can make career changes
- It shapes your financial flexibility early in your career

Many students focus on the outcome—a stable, six-figure salary.

Fewer fully understand the path it takes to get there.

RESIDENCY IS NOT ALWAYS **Optional**

If you are interested in becoming a Clinical Pharmacist, residency is often part of the equation.

- **PGY1** builds general clinical skills
- **PGY2** opens doors to specialized practice

Not every pharmacist completes a residency.

But many of the most competitive clinical roles either require it—or strongly prefer it.

This creates a reality that surprises many students:

Graduating with a PharmD may not be the final step.

It may be the beginning of another phase of training.

That has implications:

- Additional years of lower income

- Increased competition
- A need for long-term planning

Retail vs Clinical — Two Very Different Careers

One of the most important distinctions in pharmacy is often not fully understood early on.

Retail pharmacy and clinical pharmacy are not simply different settings.

They are fundamentally different experiences.

Retail pharmacy often involves:

- High prescription volume
- Time pressure
- Constant interruptions
- Customer-facing interactions
- Insurance and workflow challenges

Clinical pharmacy often involves:

- Medication optimization
- Collaboration with healthcare teams
- Complex decision-making
- Less direct patient volume, but higher responsibility per decision

Both paths require skill.

Both have value.

But they feel very different day to day.

Understanding which environment aligns with your personality is critical.

The Day-to-Day Is Not What You Think

Many students are drawn to pharmacy because they enjoy science, medications, and problem-solving.

Those elements are part of the role.

But the day-to-day reality often includes:

- Reviewing and verifying orders

- Navigating systems and workflows
- Managing interruptions
- Maintaining accuracy over long periods

The work is meaningful.

But it is also structured, repetitive at times, and detail-driven.

If you are expecting constant variation or high-visibility patient interaction, the reality may feel different than expected.

You Will Be Responsible—and **Often Unseen**

As your reflection captured, one of the defining characteristics of this role is the balance between responsibility and visibility.

You will:

- Prevent errors
- Improve care
- Influence outcomes

And many of those contributions will not be publicly recognized.

For some people, this is perfectly acceptable.

For others, it can become a source of frustration over time.

Knowing how much visibility and recognition matter to you is part of making the right decision.

The Cognitive Load **Is a Lifestyle**

Clinical pharmacy is mentally demanding.

Not occasionally—consistently.

The role requires:

- Sustained focus
- Attention to detail
- Continuous evaluation of risk

There is very little margin for inattention.

This creates a form of fatigue that is not always visible—but is very real.

Some people thrive in this type of environment.

Others find it draining over time.

Understanding how you respond to sustained mental effort is essential.

The System Will Frustrate You

Healthcare systems are complex.

And they do not always allow for ideal decisions.

You may encounter:

- Insurance limitations
- Formulary restrictions
- Medication shortages
- Administrative barriers

You may know the best option for a patient—and still not be able to implement it.

This creates tension.

And how you handle that tension matters.

There Are Exceptional Opportunities—But They Are Earned

Pharmacy offers strong career paths.

Specialization, leadership, industry roles, and advanced clinical positions are all possible.

But they are not automatic.

They require:

- Strategic decisions early in your career
- Additional training or certification
- Consistent effort and growth

The degree opens the door.

What you do after that determines where you go.

Alignment Matters More Than Prestige

It is easy to choose a career based on:

- Stability
- Income

- Reputation

But those factors alone do not determine long-term satisfaction.

Using Mason's Alignment Theory (MAT), and applying:

- **PACES™** (Personality, Aptitude, Constraints, Experience, Situation)
- **CARESET™** (Culture, Autonomy, Resources, Expectations, Environment, Team)

You can evaluate whether this role fits you.

Not just whether you can succeed in it.

Because many people are capable of becoming pharmacists.

Fewer are aligned with the day-to-day reality of the work.

What Smart Students **Do Differently**

Students who make confident, informed decisions tend to do a few things differently:

- They shadow in multiple settings (retail, hospital, specialty)
- They talk to practicing pharmacists—not just advisors
- They ask about workflow, not just responsibilities
- They explore both the positive and challenging aspects of the role
- They consider long-term fit—not just short-term outcomes

They do not rely on assumptions.

They seek clarity.

The Honest Takeaway

Pharmacy is a meaningful, impactful, and respected profession.

It offers stability, intellectual challenge, and the opportunity to make a real difference in patient care.

But it also requires:

- A significant investment
- A tolerance for sustained mental workload
- Comfort with structured systems
- Acceptance of limited visibility in many settings

There is no universal answer.

Only the answer that fits you.

And the more clearly you understand the reality now—

The more confident, intentional, and aligned your decision will be moving forward.

34

SHORTAGE SIGNAL™

Market Demand, Workforce Trends, and What It Means for You

You will hear the word "shortage" often in healthcare.

Nursing shortage.

Physician shortage.

Pharmacist shortage.

But the reality is more nuanced than a single word.

This section is designed to help you understand what is actually happening in the pharmacy workforce—so you can interpret demand correctly and make smarter, more informed career decisions.

What People Mean When They Say "Shortage"

In simple terms, a shortage suggests that there are more open roles than there are qualified professionals to fill them.

But in healthcare, the concept is rarely that straightforward.

A perceived shortage can be influenced by:

- Geographic distribution
- Practice setting
- Experience requirements
- Organizational structure

In some areas, there may be a high demand for pharmacists.

In others, the market may feel competitive or even saturated.

The key is understanding that demand is not uniform.

The Reality in Pharmacy — It Depends on Where You Look

Pharmacy does not operate as a single, unified job market.

Different settings experience demand very differently.

Retail Pharmacy:

- Often has consistent demand
- Higher turnover in some environments
- Ongoing need for licensed pharmacists

Hospital and Clinical Pharmacy:

- More competitive in many regions
- Frequently requires residency or prior experience
- Fewer positions relative to applicants

Specialty and Advanced Roles:

- Growing demand in areas like oncology, ambulatory care, and specialty pharmacy
- Often require additional training or certification

This creates an important distinction:

There may be demand in the profession...

But not necessarily in every role, setting, or location.

Why the Market Can Feel Tight

Even when there is demand, it may not feel that way to new graduates or those seeking specific roles.

Several factors contribute to this:

Residency Bottlenecks:

Clinical roles often prefer or require residency training, which limits access for those without it.

Experience Expectations:

Employers may seek candidates who are already familiar with their systems or workflows.

Geographic Preferences:

Many candidates target the same regions or institutions, increasing competition.

Workflow and Organizational Design:

Some organizations structure roles in ways that limit hiring, even when workloads are high.

These factors can create the perception that opportunities are limited—even when they exist.

Turnover vs. True Shortage

In some settings, especially high-volume environments, demand is driven by turnover rather than expansion.

This distinction matters.

- **Turnover-driven demand** means roles are frequently open—but may come with challenging conditions.
- **Growth-driven demand** suggests expanding opportunities and evolving roles.

Understanding the difference helps you evaluate not just whether a job is available—but whether it is a role you actually want.

The Misalignment Factor

One of the most important—and often overlooked—drivers of workforce instability is misalignment.

Using Mason's Alignment Theory (MAT), and applying:

- **PACES™** (Personality, Aptitude, Constraints, Experience, Situation)
- **CARESET™** (Culture, Autonomy, Resources, Expectations, Environment, Team)

we can see that:

Many workforce challenges are not simply about supply.

They are about fit.

When roles:

- Do not match how people are wired
- Require sustained conditions that are difficult to maintain
- Create environments where professionals feel unsupported

people leave.

This creates ongoing demand—not because there are not enough trained professionals, but because the roles themselves are difficult to sustain.

What This Means for You

Understanding workforce trends is not just about predicting job availability.

It is about making strategic decisions.

As you consider this path, ask:

- Where is demand strongest—and why?
- What qualifications are expected for the roles I want?
- Am I willing to relocate or adapt to different settings?
- Does the environment associated with high demand align with me?

A role being "in demand" does not automatically make it a good fit.

And a competitive role does not make it out of reach—if you plan intentionally.

The Long-Term Outlook

Several factors continue to shape the future of pharmacy:

Aging Population:

Increased medication use and chronic disease management will sustain demand for medication expertise.

Specialty Medications:

Growth in complex therapies requires specialized knowledge and monitoring.

Technology and Automation:

Some tasks are becoming more efficient—but clinical judgment remains essential.

Expanded Roles:

Pharmacists are increasingly involved in direct patient care, chronic disease management, and team-based healthcare.

The profession is evolving.

But not all roles are evolving in the same way.

Signal vs. Noise

It is easy to be influenced by headlines, statistics, or generalized statements about workforce trends.

But the most important signals are often more specific:

- The needs of a particular setting
- The expectations of a specific role
- The culture of an individual organization

Pay attention to those signals.

They will tell you far more about your potential experience than broad industry narratives.

The Honest Takeaway

There is opportunity in pharmacy.

But it is not evenly distributed.

Some paths are more accessible.

Some are more competitive.

Some are more sustainable than others.

Understanding these differences allows you to:

- Set realistic expectations
- Make strategic decisions
- Choose paths that align with both your goals and your environment

Because success in this field is not just about entering the profession.

It is about finding the right place within it.

35

THE CAREER TRAP™

When a "Good Career" Quietly Becomes the Wrong One

One of the most dangerous outcomes in a health-care career is not failure.

It is success... in the wrong role.

Because when a career looks stable, respected, and financially secure, it becomes much harder to question—even when it no longer feels right.

This is what we call **The Career Trap™**.

And it shows up more often in pharmacy than most people expect.

How the Trap Begins

The path into pharmacy is structured and logical.

You:

- Complete your prerequisites
- Enter pharmacy school
- Graduate with a respected degree
- Pass your boards

- Secure a stable, well-paying job

From the outside, everything looks like it worked.

And in many ways, it did.

But the trap doesn't begin with a bad decision.

It begins with a **good decision that was never fully examined.**

A decision based on:

- Stability
- Income
- Reputation
- Practicality

All valid reasons.

But not always complete ones.

When Alignment Was Never the Question

Most people entering pharmacy never ask:

👉 "Does this fit how I am wired?"

They ask:

- "Can I get in?"
- "Can I pass?"
- "Will it pay well?"

And because they *can* do all of those things...

They move forward.

This is where misalignment begins—not from inability, but from **unexamined capability.**

The Early Years Mask the Problem

In the first 1–3 years, the Career Trap™ is almost invisible.

You are:

- Learning
- Adapting
- Building confidence

Everything feels new.

The workload feels like part of the process.

The stress feels temporary.

And because you are progressing, you assume:

👉 "This is just what it takes."

And sometimes, it is.

But sometimes, it isn't.

When the Questions Start Showing Up

Around years 3–5, something shifts.

Not dramatically.

Quietly.

You begin to notice:

- The work doesn't energize you the way you expected
- Certain parts of the job feel heavier than they should
- The pace or structure feels harder to sustain

And the question appears:

👉 "Is this just part of the job... or is this not the right fit?"

This is the moment most people ignore.

Why People Stay (Even When It Doesn't Fit)

Once you are in the role, several forces make it difficult to leave:

1. Financial Commitment

Student loans create pressure to stay.

2. Identity

You didn't just get a job—you became a pharmacist.

3. External Validation

From family, peers, and society.

4. Lack of Clear Alternatives

You know this path—but not necessarily others.

So instead of reevaluating...

Most people **adapt**.

Adaptation vs. Alignment

Adaptation is powerful.

Humans can adjust to almost anything.

But adaptation is not the same as alignment.

You can:

- Perform well
- Earn well
- Be respected

And still feel:

- Drained
- Disconnected
- Unsure long-term

This is the core of The Career Trap™:

👉 **Success without fit**

What the Trap Feels Like Over Time

It rarely looks dramatic.

It looks like:

- Going through the motions
- Counting shifts instead of engaging in them
- Feeling relief when you're off—more than satisfaction when you're working
- Wondering how long you can realistically continue

Nothing is "wrong."

But something is off.

The Cost of Staying Too Long

The longer someone stays in a misaligned role, the harder it becomes to change.

Not because it's impossible.

But because:

- Financial responsibilities increase
- Lifestyle becomes tied to income
- Confidence in other paths decreases

And slowly, the question changes from:

☞ "Is this right for me?"

to

☞ "Is it too late to change?"

How to Avoid the Career Trap™

You don't avoid the trap by making perfect decisions.

You avoid it by making **aware decisions**.

That means:

- Evaluating fit early
- Paying attention to friction
- Being honest about what energizes vs drains you
- Understanding that capability ≠ alignment

And most importantly:

☞ Giving yourself permission to question a "good" path

If You're Already in It

If you're reading this and recognizing parts of your experience, you are not stuck.

You are aware.

And awareness is the starting point for change.

That change might look like:

- Adjusting your setting
- Changing your schedule
- Specializing
- Pivoting into a new area

Or simply redefining how you approach your current role.

The Honest Takeaway

The goal of a career is not just stability.

It is sustainability.

Pharmacy can absolutely provide:

- Income
- Respect
- Opportunity

But none of those guarantee alignment.

And the earlier you recognize that...

The more control you have over where your path leads next.

36

ALIGNMENT AND REFLECTION

How to Use *The Alignment Check*

The Alignment Check — 10 Questions That Matter Most is your personal pause button. It's designed to help you translate what you've just read into something real — your own clarity, curiosity, and next steps.

Think of it as a guided mirror: instead of telling you who to be, it helps you notice what already fits and what doesn't. Use it slowly, honestly, and without judgment. There are no right answers — only revealing ones.

Before You Begin

1 **Find quiet.** You'll get more from this reflection if you give it space.

2 **Keep a notebook or your phone nearby.** Jot your thoughts without editing; the rawest notes often hold the truth.

3 **Read one role at a time.** Don't rush through multiple SCRUB*fit*™ profiles. Let each one breathe.

. . .

How to Work Through the 10 Questions

• **After each profile or category,** reread *The Alignment Check* slowly, question by question.

• **Highlight what resonates.** If a question makes your heart beat faster — that's a sign of alignment. If it makes you sigh or hesitate — that's a signal, too.

• **Circle your top three responses.** These are your "alignment anchors." They point toward careers, settings, or values that match who you are.

• **Revisit the list later.** Your answers may shift as your experiences grow; alignment is a moving target, not a fixed destination.

When to Use It

• **Early exploration:** When you're still figuring out which healthcare roles fit you best.

• **Career transition:** When burnout, boredom, or curiosity says, "Maybe it's time for something different."

• **Realignment check-in:** Every six months, take five minutes to reread your answers and see what's changed.

Why It Matters

The Alignment Check helps bridge the gap between who you are and where you belong. It turns passive reading into active discovery — transforming information into insight, and insight into alignment.

The Alignment Check — 10 Questions That Matter Most

1 What first drew you to this career — curiosity, compassion, or circumstance?

2 Which part of this role feels like *you at your best*?

3 Which part would likely test your patience, endurance, or alignment?

4 How does this profession match your values, pace, and preferred kind of pressure?

5 Could you see yourself thriving in the environments where this role usually works — and why or why not?

6 What skills or experiences could you start developing right now to move closer to this path?

7 Who in your life models the professionalism or calm you'd want to bring to this career?

8 If you shadowed someone in this field for a day, what would you hope to learn about their mindset?

9 How would success in this career *feel* — not just look — in your everyday life?

10 After reading this section, does this role feel aligned, misaligned, or somewhere in between — and what does that tell you about your next step?

37

MICRO-FIT ASSESSMENT

Micro-Fit Assessment — Pharmacist

*(SCRUB*fit*™ Career Alignment Snapshot)*

Are You Aligned With the Pharmacist Path?

Pharmacists are the guardians of safe medication use, the educators behind every prescription, and the bridge between evidence and empathy.

This short 15-question self-assessment will help you see whether your personality, mindset, and values align with the pharmacy profession — whether in hospitals, retail, clinical, or research settings.

It's not about memorizing drug names — it's about recognizing if you're wired for detail, safety, and stewardship.

Answer honestly, and notice what resonates most.

Instructions

For each statement below, rate how true it feels for you on a scale of **1–10:**

1 = Not at all true **10 = Completely true**

Circle or note your number beside each statement, then total your score at the end.

Questions

1 I feel most confident when I'm trusted with precise, high- stakes responsibilities.

2 I enjoy solving problems through logic, science, and careful reasoning.

3 I find meaning in ensuring patient safety and preventing medication errors.

4 I'm energized by continuous learning — especially about new drugs and therapies.

5 I take pride in accuracy and consistency, even when no one's watching.

6 I feel fulfilled when patients understand their medications and feel safe using them.

7 I'm comfortable managing complex details while staying calm under pressure.

8 I enjoy collaborating with nurses, physicians, and other clinicians to improve care.

9 I'm naturally methodical — I prefer double-checking over rushing.

10 I like connecting science to human stories — the "why" behind every prescription.

11 I believe that ethics and responsibility are as important as knowledge.

12 I find satisfaction in maintaining order, documentation, and safety standards.

13 I'm drawn to a role where precision directly affects patient outcomes.

14 I recover quickly from long hours because I find purpose in doing things right.

15 I want a career that combines intellect, empathy, and integrity every single day.

SCORING GUIDE

Add your scores for all 15 statements.

Your total will place you in one of three alignment zones:

Total Points

Alignment Zone

Interpretation

120–150

High Alignment

You're wired for the pharmacy world — precise, ethical, and committed to excellence. You likely belong in *The Med Heads* SCRUB*fit*™ category.

90–119

Partial Alignment

You share many Pharmacist traits — detail-oriented, analytical, caring — but may thrive in related areas like **The Vital Link** or **The Diagnostic Division.**

Below 90

Misalignment Zone

Your values or energy may align better with another role. That's clarity, not failure — explore where your rhythm fits best.

REFLECTION PROMPT

Circle or highlight the three statements that made you pause — either because they felt deeply true or surprisingly uncertain.

Ask yourself:

"Do I find peace in precision, or pressure?"

Your answer reveals where your alignment lives.

. . .

Next Step

For a deeper, personalized look at your alignment across all 21 *SCRUB*fit*™* roles, take the complete **SCRUB*fit*™ Healthcare Career Assessment** at **SCRUBfit.club.**

Use **Promo Code: smart** for **25% off** your assessment.

Because the opposite of alignment isn't failure — it's a miserable life.

Choose alignment. Thrive in your calling.

Love every minute of your career as a Pharmacist.

38

BEFORE YOU COMMIT

What Most Future Pharmacists Don't Think About

Choosing to become a Pharmacist is often framed as a logical decision.

It's stable.

It's respected.

It's financially viable.

And on paper, all of that is true.

But what most people don't fully explore before committing to this path is what the work actually feels like—day after day, year after year.

Because a career is not just defined by what it offers.

It is defined by what it requires.

What Does the Work Feel Like Every Day?

Before committing to pharmacy, it's important to move beyond the surface-level understanding of the role.

Ask yourself:

- Can I stay mentally focused for long periods without losing precision?
- Am I comfortable making decisions where small errors can have serious consequences?

• Do I find satisfaction in detail-oriented work, even when it feels repetitive?

Pharmacy is not just knowledge—it is sustained attention.

If you thrive in environments that require constant accuracy and vigilance, the work can feel engaging.

If you don't, it can feel draining very quickly.

Am I Comfortable With Responsibility That Doesn't Turn Off?

One of the realities of pharmacy is that responsibility does not always end when your shift does.

You may go home and:

• Replay decisions

• Wonder if something was missed

• Mentally revisit complex cases

This is not constant—but it happens.

And for some people, it's manageable.

For others, it becomes exhausting.

Understanding how you carry responsibility is critical before stepping into a role that requires it consistently.

Do I Need Recognition — or Am I Comfortable Being Behind the Scenes?

Pharmacy is a profession where much of your impact is invisible.

You prevent problems more often than you solve them in front of others.

You may:

• Catch an error that no one else noticed

• Adjust a dose that avoids complications

• Make a recommendation that quietly improves care

And many of these moments will go unrecognized.

If you need consistent external validation, this can feel frustrating.

If you find satisfaction in the work itself, it becomes sustainable.

What Kind of Pace Fits Me Best?

Pharmacy exists across a wide range of environments, each with a different pace.

Some roles are:

- Fast, unpredictable, and high-pressure
- Steady, structured, and routine-based
- Analytical, slow-moving, and detail-heavy

No single pace is better than another.

But one will fit you better.

Choosing the wrong pace is one of the fastest ways to feel misaligned—even in a role you are fully capable of performing.

How Do I Handle Interruptions and Constant Task Switching?

In many pharmacy settings, especially clinical and hospital roles, interruptions are part of the workflow.

You may be:

- Verifying an order
- Interrupted by a nurse question
- Pulled into a clinical discussion
- Returning to your original task

This happens repeatedly throughout the day.

If you can shift focus quickly and re-engage without losing accuracy, you will adapt well.

If constant interruptions break your concentration, the environment may feel overwhelming.

Am I Okay With the Mental Load of Precision Work?

Pharmacy requires a level of attention that does not fluctuate with mood or energy.

Even on days when you feel tired or distracted, the expectation remains the same:

Be accurate.

Be thorough.

Be responsible.

This consistency is what protects patients.

But it also requires discipline.

Understanding whether you can sustain that level of focus is essential.

How Important Is Flexibility in My Life?

Depending on your role, pharmacy can limit flexibility.

This may include:

- Fixed schedules
- Weekend or holiday shifts
- Limited ability to step away during the day

Some roles offer more control than others, but all come with structure.

If flexibility is a top priority, this is something to evaluate carefully.

Am I Drawn to the Work — or the Idea of the Work?

This is one of the most important questions to ask.

Many people are drawn to pharmacy because of what it represents:

- Stability
- Professional identity
- Financial security

But the reality of the work is different from the idea of it.

Take the time to understand:

- The daily tasks
- The pace
- The expectations

Because long-term satisfaction comes from the experience—not the perception.

Can I See Myself Doing This Repeatedly?

Not just once.

Not just in training.

But repeatedly.

Day after day.

Pharmacy is built on consistency.

If the core tasks feel tolerable but not engaging, that feeling will compound over time.

If they feel meaningful, even in small ways, that meaning will grow.

What Happens If I Realize It's Not the Right Fit?

This is not a question people ask often—but they should.

The truth is:

Pharmacy is not one path.

It is many.

If one setting does not fit, there are others:

- Clinical
- Ambulatory
- Industry
- Specialty
- Long-term care
- Data and safety roles

Changing direction is not failure.

It is alignment.

Understanding that flexibility exists reduces pressure and opens options.

The Decision Most People Don't Realize They're Making

When you choose pharmacy, you are not just choosing a career.

You are choosing:

- A type of thinking
- A level of responsibility
- A daily experience

The question is not:

👉 "Can I do this?"

The question is:

👉 "Does this fit how I want to live and work every day?"

Because capability gets you into the profession.

Alignment is what keeps you there.

Final Thought

Pharmacy can be an incredibly rewarding career.

It offers stability, purpose, and the opportunity to make a real impact.

But it also requires clarity.

The more honest you are with yourself before committing, the more likely you are to find a path that works—not just in theory, but in reality.

And that is what ultimately determines whether this becomes a career you endure...

Or one you can truly sustain.

39

THE LONG GAME

What a Career in Pharmacy Really Becomes Over Time

When most people think about becoming a Pharmacist, they think about the beginning.

Getting into school.

Passing boards.

Landing that first job.

But what they don't think about—and what ultimately matters more—is what the career becomes over time.

Because pharmacy is not a single decision.

It is a long sequence of decisions, adjustments, realizations, and pivots that shape not just your work, but your life.

And the way it unfolds is rarely what you expect at the start.

The First Phase — Proving You Can Do It

Early in your career, everything is about capability.

You are focused on:

- Getting it right
- Building confidence
- Learning how the real world actually works

Every decision feels heavier because it's new. Every interaction requires effort. You are constantly thinking, constantly checking, constantly trying to keep up.

This phase is intense—but necessary.

It's where you build the foundation:

- Clinical judgment
- Workflow awareness
- Communication skills

You are not just learning pharmacy.

You are learning how to be responsible for it.

And for most people, this phase is the hardest.

The Second Phase — Becoming Reliable

At some point, something shifts.

The work doesn't become easy—but it becomes familiar.

You begin to:

- Recognize patterns faster
- Make decisions more confidently
- Communicate more clearly

You are no longer proving you can do the job.

You are becoming someone others rely on.

This is where your role starts to expand—even if your title doesn't.

People come to you with questions.

They trust your judgment.

They expect consistency.

And this is where many pharmacists settle into their careers.

Stable. Capable. Respected.

But not always fulfilled.

The Third Phase — Questioning the Fit

This is the phase that most people don't anticipate.

Once you know you can do the work, a different question begins to surface:

👉 "Do I want to keep doing this?"

Not because you can't.

But because you now understand what it requires.

This is where alignment becomes unavoidable.

You begin to notice:

- What parts of the job give you energy
- What parts drain you consistently
- What feels sustainable—and what doesn't

For some, the answer is clear:

"This fits. I'm in the right place."

For others, it's more complicated.

"This works... but something feels off."

And this is where many people get stuck.

Because the job is "good."

But good is not the same as aligned.

The Fourth Phase — Adjusting or Pivoting

This is where the most important decisions happen.

Not at the beginning of your career.

But here.

You have options:

- Stay and adjust how you work
- Shift roles within your current environment
- Move into a different pharmacy setting
- Transition into a new path entirely

What matters is not the direction itself.

It is the intention behind it.

The pharmacists who sustain long careers are not the ones who picked perfectly at the start.

They are the ones who adjusted when they needed to.

The Fifth Phase — Building a Career That Fits

Over time, if you stay aware and willing to adapt, something changes.

The work begins to feel different.

Not because it is easier.

But because it fits.

You understand:

- Where you perform best
- What environments suit you
- How to manage your energy

You stop trying to force yourself into roles that don't work.

And you start choosing roles that do.

This is where sustainability happens.

Not by accident.

But by design.

What Most People Get Wrong

Many people approach pharmacy like a one-time decision.

Pick the right path.

Commit.

Stay.

But that's not how it works.

The real skill is not choosing perfectly at the beginning.

It is staying aware throughout the process.

Because what fits you at 25 may not fit you at 35.

What energizes you early in your career may drain you later.

And that's not failure.

That's evolution.

The Hidden Advantage of Pharmacy

One of the greatest strengths of this profession is its flexibility—once you understand how to use it.

Pharmacy is not one lane.

It is many:

- Clinical
- Ambulatory
- Industry
- Specialty
- Data and safety
- Leadership

Each offers a different experience.

A different pace.

A different type of thinking.

A different lifestyle.

And that means you are not locked in.

You are positioned.

The Real Goal

The goal is not to find a perfect job.

The goal is to build a career that works for you over time.

A career where:

- The demands are manageable
- The work feels meaningful
- The lifestyle is sustainable

That does not happen by default.

It happens through awareness and adjustment.

Final Perspective

If you choose pharmacy, you are choosing a profession that will challenge you.

It will ask for:

- Precision
- Discipline
- Responsibility

But it will also give you something in return:

The ability to make a real difference.

Quietly. Consistently. Meaningfully.

The key is not just getting into the profession.

It is staying in it in a way that works.

Because a career is not defined by how it starts.

It is defined by how well it fits—over time.

40

THE REALITY CHECK

What This Career Demands Over 10, 20, and 30 Years

No one talks about what this career feels like over decades.

They talk about getting in.

They talk about getting through school.

They talk about getting the job.

But they don't talk about staying.

And staying is where everything changes.

Because pharmacy is not just something you do.

It is something you carry.

Year 1–3 — Survival and Proving Ground

In the beginning, everything feels intense.

You are thinking constantly.

Checking everything.

Second-guessing yourself more than you admit.

Even simple decisions take effort because they are new.

Even routine tasks feel heavy because they matter.

You are building:

- your clinical judgment
- your workflow rhythm

• your confidence

And it's exhausting.

Not because you're failing.

But because you are growing into responsibility that didn't exist before.

This phase is where many people quietly wonder:

👉 "Did I make the right decision?"

And the truth is—this phase is not the career.

It's the entry point.

Year 3–7 — Competence and Expectation

At some point, things click.

You stop thinking about every step.

You start recognizing patterns.

You move faster—but more importantly, you move with clarity.

Now people trust you.

They expect you to:

• know what you're doing
• catch what others miss
• handle pressure without hesitation

This is where your identity as a pharmacist solidifies.

But this is also where something new appears:

Expectation without relief.

You are no longer being evaluated.

You are being relied on.

And that shift carries weight.

Year 7–15 — The Fork in the Road

This is where the career becomes personal.

Because now you know:

• what the job is
• what it takes
• what it costs

And a new question shows up:

👉 "Is this how I want to keep living?"

Not because the job is bad.

But because you now understand it fully.

This is where pharmacists split into different paths:

• Those who are aligned → they stay and grow

• Those who are misaligned → they feel stuck but capable

And this is where burnout begins for many.

Not from inability.

From misfit.

Year 15–25 — Adjustment or Accumulation

At this stage, you either:

👉 adjust your path

or

👉 accumulate frustration

There is no neutral.

If you stay in a role that does not fit:

• the work feels heavier

• the days feel longer

• the meaning fades

If you adjust:

• the work stabilizes

• your energy returns

• your perspective shifts

This is where alignment becomes non-negotiable.

Because you can't outwork misalignment forever.

Year 25+ — Sustainability or Exit

At this point, the outcome is clear.

You either:

• built a career that works

or

• stayed in one that didn't

The pharmacists who remain engaged this long did one thing differently:

👉 They adjusted when they needed to

Not dramatically.

But intentionally.

They:

• changed settings

- changed pace
- changed expectations

They didn't force themselves to fit the role.

They found roles that fit them.

What No One Tells You About Longevity

Longevity in pharmacy is not about endurance.

It's about alignment.

The people who last are not:

- the smartest
- the fastest
- the most driven

They are the ones who figured out:

👉 how they work best

👉 where they function best

👉 what they can sustain

And they built around that.

The Cost of Ignoring This

If you ignore alignment, the cost shows up slowly.

Not in failure.

In friction.

You feel:

- more tired than you should
- more frustrated than expected
- less connected to the work

And you start telling yourself:

👉 "This is just how it is."

It's not.

That's the most dangerous assumption in this profession.

The Advantage You Have Right Now

If you're reading this before fully committing—or early in your career—you have something incredibly valuable:

Awareness.

You know:

- what the job really feels like
- what it demands

• what it costs

Most people don't get that until years in.

That awareness gives you leverage.

You can:

• choose better

• adjust sooner

• avoid staying stuck

The Career Is Not the Job

This is the most important distinction.

Your job is where you are right now.

Your career is the path you build over time.

If your current role doesn't fit, that does not mean:

👉 "Pharmacy isn't for me"

It may mean:

👉 "This version of pharmacy isn't for me"

And that difference matters.

The Long Game Decision

At the end of the day, this is the decision you are making:

Not:

👉 "Can I do this?"

But:

👉 "Can I live this?"

Because pharmacy is not something you visit.

It's something you repeat.

Day after day.

Year after year.

And the only way that works long-term is if:

👉 the work fits who you are

Not perfectly.

But well enough to sustain.

Final Reality

Pharmacy will give you:

• stability

• responsibility

• impact

But it will also require:

- focus
- discipline
- consistency

The people who succeed long-term are not the ones who ignore that tradeoff.

They are the ones who understand it—and build a career that balances it.

That's the difference between surviving this profession...

and actually staying in it.

41

INTELLIGENT INTERVIEWS™

Walking into an interview for a Clinical Pharmacist role is very different from most traditional job interviews. This is not simply a conversation about your background, your strengths, or your interest in the position. It is an evaluation of how you think, how you make decisions under pressure, and how you operate when patient safety is on the line. Employers are not just hiring your knowledge—they are assessing your judgment.

Clinical Pharmacist interviews are designed to test both your clinical competence and your professional presence. You may be asked to walk through real-world scenarios, interpret lab values, evaluate medication regimens, or explain how you would handle a potential medication error. These questions are not meant to trick you, but they are meant to reveal how you approach complex problems. The goal is not perfection. The goal is to demonstrate a safe, thoughtful, and structured approach.

Preparation for these interviews requires more than reviewing drug information. You need to understand how to communicate your thinking clearly and confidently. When presented with a scenario, slow down just enough to structure your response. Identify the key clinical concerns, explain your reasoning, and outline your recommendation. Even if you are unsure of the exact answer, showing a safe and logical thought process is often more important than arriving at a perfect conclusion.

One of the most important skills you can demonstrate is the ability to prioritize. In real clinical environments, you will often be balancing multiple demands at once. Interviewers want to see that you can identify what matters most and act accordingly. When answering questions, make it clear how you would triage competing priorities and ensure that high-risk situations are addressed first.

Communication is another critical component. Clinical Pharmacists serve as a bridge between providers, nurses, and patients. During the interview, your ability to explain complex information in a clear and concise way is being evaluated at all times. Avoid overly technical language when it is not necessary, and focus on clarity. The strongest candidates are those who can translate clinical knowledge into practical, actionable guidance.

You should also expect behavioral questions that explore how you have handled situations in the past. These may include times when you caught an error, disagreed with a provider, or worked through a challenging patient case. When answering these questions, focus on the impact of your actions. What did you identify? What did you do? What was the outcome? Employers are looking for evidence that you can operate effectively in real-world conditions.

Another area that is often overlooked is how you present your mindset. Clinical Pharmacists are expected to be both confident and collaborative. Overconfidence can come across as dismissive, while lack of confidence can raise concerns about decision-making. The goal is to demonstrate that you are thoughtful, open to input, and committed to patient safety above all else.

Research is a non-negotiable part of interview preparation. You should have a clear understanding of the organization, its patient population, and its clinical focus areas. If you are interviewing at a hospital, know their specialties, recent initiatives, and any publicly available information about quality or safety outcomes. If you are interviewing in a specialized area such as oncology or critical care, be prepared to speak to relevant clinical considerations.

It is also important to understand the workflow and expectations of the role you are applying for. Not all Clinical Pharmacist positions are the same. Some are heavily operational, others are more clinical, and some blend both. Asking thoughtful questions about daily responsibilities, team structure, and expectations shows that you are evaluating fit just as much as they are evaluating you.

Working with a recruiter or hiring manager requires professionalism and responsiveness. Communication should be timely, clear, and respectful. Small details matter. How you handle scheduling, follow-up, and general correspondence can influence how you are perceived as a candidate.

After the interview, follow-up is not optional—it is expected. A brief, professional message expressing appreciation for the opportunity reinforces your interest and professionalism. It also keeps you top of mind as decisions are being made. In healthcare environments where collaboration and communication are essential, these small signals carry weight.

Ultimately, the Clinical Pharmacist interview is not about proving that you know everything. It is about demonstrating that you can think critically, communicate effectively, and prioritize patient safety in every situation. Employers are looking for someone they can trust —not just with knowledge, but with judgment.

If you approach the interview with preparation, structure, and a clear focus on safety and collaboration, you position yourself as a candidate who is ready not just to do the job, but to do it well.

42

THE FINAL FIT CHECK

Before You Step Into Pharmacy

Before someone commits to pharmacy, they need more than encouragement. They need honesty. This profession can offer stability, purpose, respect, and meaningful impact, but it also requires a very specific kind of person to sustain it well. Pharmacy is not simply a career for people who like science. It is a career for people who can carry precision, responsibility, and patience across thousands of small decisions without losing sight of the human being behind each one.

The final question is not whether pharmacy is a good profession. It is. The better question is whether pharmacy is a good fit for you. That distinction matters because a role can be respected, well-paid, and important while still being misaligned with how someone thinks, works, and lives. A person can be capable of doing the work and still find the daily experience draining. Capability gets you through training, but alignment determines whether you can stay.

Start by asking how you respond to responsibility. In pharmacy, the consequences of your work are not theoretical. A missed interaction, a dosing error, an overlooked allergy alert (gl), or a rushed verification can matter. This does not mean you need to be fearful. It means you need to respect the weight of the role. The best pharmacists are not careless optimists or anxious perfectionists. They are disciplined professionals who understand that safety is built through consistent habits.

Next, ask how you handle repetition. Much of pharmacy involves repeated actions: reviewing orders, checking doses, confirming routes of administration (gl), documenting interventions, counseling patients, and verifying accuracy. To someone outside the field, repetition may look simple. Inside the profession, repetition is where vigilance is tested. The work may look familiar, but the patient behind the work is never generic. You have to bring fresh attention to tasks that may appear routine.

You should also understand your relationship with interruptions. Pharmacy rarely unfolds in a perfectly quiet sequence. A nurse may call while you are reviewing a high-alert medication (gl). A provider may ask for clarification while you are documenting a medication reconciliation (gl). A patient may need counseling while the queue continues to build. If you lose accuracy every time your attention shifts, certain pharmacy environments may feel punishing. If you can pause, anchor your place, respond, and return safely, you may adapt well.

Another fit question involves visibility. Many pharmacists do some of their most important work behind the scenes. They prevent harm that no one ever sees. They correct orders before they become errors. They clarify instructions before confusion reaches the patient. They support the care team without always receiving public recognition. If you need applause to feel useful, pharmacy may frustrate you. If quiet impact matters to you, the work can feel deeply meaningful.

You also need to consider the emotional shape of the profession. Pharmacy is not emotionless just because it is precise. A pediatric dose, an oncology regimen, a controlled substance (gl) concern, or an adverse drug reaction (gl) report can carry real emotional weight. The pharmacist may not always be the person holding the patient's hand, but the pharmacist is still part of the patient's story. The emotional work is often quieter, but it is not absent.

Financially, pharmacy should be evaluated with clear eyes. The salary may look strong, but the educational investment can be significant. Student loans, interest, licensing, continuing education, and professional costs all affect the real return. A career is not automatically financially healthy because the income is respectable. The full picture includes debt, lifestyle, schedule, and long-term flexibility.

You should also think about what kind of pharmacy environment fits your energy. A hospital pharmacist may thrive on interdisciplinary teamwork and acute decision-making. A community pharmacist may find purpose in relationships and patient access. A clinical pharmacist may enjoy rounding, medication therapy decisions, and complex care planning. An informatics pharmacist may prefer systems, data, and technology. A pharmacovigilance pharmacist may find meaning in signal detection and medication safety patterns. These are not interchangeable lives. They are different versions of the profession.

This is where Mason's Alignment Theory (MAT) matters. PACES™ and CARESET™ help move the decision beyond "Can I become a pharmacist?" and into "Which version of pharmacy fits me best?" Your Personality, Aptitude, Constraints, Experience, and Situation shape how the work feels. The Culture, Autonomy, Resources, Expectations, Structure, Environment, and Team around you shape whether the role becomes sustainable. A strong pharmacist in the wrong environment can still burn out. A well-aligned pharmacist in the right environment can build a long, meaningful career.

Before you commit, pay attention to what gives you energy. Do you enjoy solving complex medication problems? Do you like explaining things clearly to patients? Do you feel satisfaction when a system becomes safer because of a process improvement? Do you prefer direct interaction, quiet analysis, teaching, leadership, or technical precision? These preferences are not minor details. They are clues.

Also pay attention to what drains you. If constant interruptions leave you exhausted, a high-volume retail environment may not be the best long-term fit. If emotional intensity overwhelms you, oncology or pediatrics may require careful consideration. If repetitive verification feels intolerable, a more clinical, consultative, or systems-based path may be better. If ambiguity frustrates you, roles with clearer protocols may suit you more than rapidly evolving specialties.

The point is not to scare anyone away from pharmacy. The point is to help people choose with accuracy. Pharmacy needs people who understand what they are entering. It needs professionals who respect the responsibility, value the details, and care enough to stay thoughtful when the work becomes routine. It also needs people who are honest about their own limits.

A sustainable pharmacy career is not built by ignoring discomfort. It is built by interpreting discomfort correctly. Sometimes discomfort means you are growing. Sometimes it means you are in the wrong setting. Sometimes it means your workload is unreasonable. Sometimes it means your role no longer fits your season of life. The earlier you can tell the difference, the better decisions you will make.

The final fit check is simple, but not easy: can you see yourself doing this work repeatedly, responsibly, and with enough meaning to stay engaged? Can you handle the precision without becoming brittle? Can you carry the responsibility without letting it consume you? Can you work within systems while still advocating for patients? Can you accept that much of your best work may be invisible?

If the answer is yes, pharmacy may offer a powerful and purposeful path. If the answer is no, that is not failure. It is information. And information, used honestly, can prevent years of misalignment.

Pharmacy is a profession of trust. Patients trust that what they receive is safe. Providers trust that recommendations are sound. Teams trust that pharmacists will notice what others miss. That trust is earned through discipline, judgment, communication, and care.

Before you step into the profession, make sure you understand not only what pharmacy asks of you, but what you need in return. The best career decision is not the one that looks most impressive from the outside. It is the one you can live with from the inside.

43

FIRST 90 DAYS AS A CLINICAL PHARMACIST

What Actually Happens

The first ninety days are not about proving you're smart.

They're about proving you're safe, consistent, and reliable in a system that depends on accuracy.

No matter how strong your academic background is, the transition into real practice introduces a different kind of pressure. You are no longer answering questions—you are responsible for outcomes. The goal in this phase is not perfection. It is stability.

Week 1 — Orientation, Systems, and Reality

Your first week is less about clinical decisions and more about learning how the environment functions.

You will be introduced to:

- the EMR (gl) and how orders flow through it
- order verification (gl) queues and prioritization
- the formulary (gl) and local protocols
- communication pathways with nurses and providers

Everything feels slower than expected. Not because the work is easy, but because every step is unfamiliar. You will double-check simple things, ask questions frequently, and rely on others more than you anticipated.

That's normal.

The biggest mistake in Week 1 is trying to move too fast. Speed comes later. Right now, accuracy is everything.

Weeks 2–4 — Supervised Decision-Making

As you move into the second and third weeks, your role begins to expand.

You start:

- verifying orders with oversight
- reviewing dosing adjustments
- identifying basic interactions
- participating in patient-specific discussions

This is where the mental load becomes real.

You are no longer just observing—you are contributing.

You will experience your first "pause moment," where something doesn't feel right. Maybe it's a dose that seems off, a duplication that shouldn't be there, or a patient profile that doesn't align with the order.

That hesitation is not weakness.

It is the beginning of clinical judgment.

Use it.

The First Near-Miss — And Why It Matters

At some point in the first month, you will encounter a situation where something almost slips through.

Maybe you catch it at the last second.

Maybe someone else points it out.

Either way, it stays with you.

This moment is important.

It reinforces:

- the importance of attention to detail
- the role of safety systems like DUR (gl)
- the value of slowing down when needed

You don't learn this from a lecture.

You learn it from experience.

And it sharpens how you approach every decision after.

Month 2 — Building Rhythm

By the second month, you begin to develop a rhythm.

You:

- move through systems more efficiently
- recognize common medication patterns
- understand workflow priorities

You are still thinking through decisions, but not from scratch every time.

Patterns start to emerge.

You'll notice:

- recurring dosing adjustments
- common therapeutic duplications (gl)
- frequent documentation expectations

This is where confidence begins—but it must be controlled.

The risk in Month 2 is not lack of knowledge.

It is premature confidence.

Stay disciplined.

Communication Becomes Critical

As your clinical role grows, so does your communication responsibility.

You will:

- clarify orders with providers
- respond to nurse questions
- document recommendations

Clarity matters.

A correct recommendation that is poorly communicated can be ignored or misunderstood. A clear, concise explanation builds trust quickly.

You are not just verifying medications.

You are becoming part of a clinical conversation.

Month 3 — From Task to Responsibility

By the third month, expectations change.

You are no longer seen as "new."

You are expected to:

- manage your workflow
- prioritize effectively
- recognize risk independently

This is where the role shifts.

You are not just completing tasks.

You are accountable for decisions.

You will still ask questions. You will still confirm uncertainties. But the responsibility is now yours to carry more consistently.

This is the turning point.

Time Management Reality

One of the biggest challenges in the first 90 days is time management.

You will feel:

- behind at times
- interrupted frequently
- pulled in multiple directions

Learning to:

- prioritize high-alert medications (gl)
- pause and anchor before switching tasks
- return to work without losing accuracy

These are skills, not instincts.

And they take time to build.

What Separates Those Who Stabilize from Those Who Struggle

By the end of 90 days, a pattern becomes clear.

Those who stabilize tend to:

- slow down when unsure
- ask focused questions
- build consistent workflows
- accept the learning curve

Those who struggle often:

- rush to keep up
- avoid asking for clarification
- rely on memory instead of process
- react instead of prioritize

The difference is not intelligence.

It is approach.

What You Should Expect to Feel

By the end of three months, you should not expect to feel "finished."

You should expect to feel:

- more aware
- more responsible
- more deliberate

You will still encounter unfamiliar situations.

You will still pause before decisions.

But those pauses become more controlled.

That is progress.

Final Perspective on the First 90 Days

The first 90 days are not about becoming an expert.

They are about becoming dependable.

If you can:

- maintain accuracy
- manage your pace
- recognize risk
- communicate clearly

You are building the foundation that everything else depends on.

Confidence will come later.

Speed will come later.

Mastery will come later.

Right now, the goal is simple:

Be safe.

Be consistent.

Be willing to learn.

Everything else builds from there.

44

WHAT CHANGES AFTER THE FIRST 90 DAYS

The First Year — What Changes After the First 90 Days

After the first 90 days, the work does not suddenly become easy. It becomes more recognizable.

That is an important difference.

You begin to understand the rhythm of the role, the personalities of the team, the pressure points in the workflow, and the situations that tend to create risk. The unfamiliar starts to become familiar. The systems that once felt overwhelming begin to feel navigable. You are still learning, but you are no longer simply trying to survive the day.

This is where the first year becomes important.

The first 90 days teach you how to function. The first year teaches you how to grow.

By month four or five, you may begin to notice that your thinking has changed. You recognize patterns faster. You know when an order deserves a second look. You understand which questions need to be asked immediately and which can wait. You begin to trust your hesitation when something feels off. That hesitation is not indecision. It is clinical instinct beginning to form.

This stage can be encouraging, but it can also be risky. As confidence grows, so does the temptation to move too quickly. You may feel pressure to prove that you no longer need help. Resist that impulse. The safest pharmacists are not the ones who stop asking questions. They are the ones who ask better questions over time.

Your first year is also when you begin building your professional reputation. People notice whether you are consistent. They notice whether your recommendations are clear. They notice whether you follow through. Nurses remember the pharmacist who responds calmly under pressure. Physicians remember the pharmacist who brings evidence instead of opinion. Colleagues remember the pharmacist who can be trusted when the queue is heavy and the day is complicated.

Reputation in pharmacy is built quietly. It is built through accuracy, communication, steadiness, and reliability. It is not built in one impressive moment. It is built through hundreds of ordinary moments handled well.

This is also when you start learning the difference between task completion and professional judgment. Early on, it can feel like success means getting through the work: verifying the orders, answering the calls, documenting the notes, completing the handoffs. But over time, you realize that completion is only part of the job. The deeper responsibility is knowing when to pause, when to question, when to escalate, and when to recommend a different path.

That is the real growth of the first year.

You also begin to understand your own limits more clearly. Some days will leave you energized. Others will leave you depleted. Pay attention to the difference. If certain tasks consistently drain you, that is information. If certain patient populations, workflows, or environments bring out your best thinking, that is information too. The first year is not only about proving yourself to the organization. It is also about learning whether this version of pharmacy fits you.

This is where many people ignore their own signals. They assume that fatigue means weakness or that frustration means they are not tough enough. Sometimes fatigue is simply part of being new. But sometimes it is a sign of misalignment. The more honest you are with yourself, the better decisions you can make.

A successful first year does not mean you never feel uncertain. It means you become safer, steadier, and more aware. You learn how to recover from hard days. You learn how to document more efficiently. You learn how to communicate without overexplaining. You learn how to admit uncertainty without losing credibility. You learn that professionalism is not pretending to know everything. It is knowing how to respond responsibly when you do not.

By the end of the first year, you should not expect to feel like you have mastered the profession. Pharmacy is too broad, too complex, and too constantly changing for that. But you should feel different than you did at the beginning. More grounded. More deliberate. More capable of seeing the whole picture.

You will still make mistakes. You will still need help. You will still encounter cases that stretch you.

But you will also begin to see yourself becoming the kind of pharmacist others can rely on.

That is the real milestone.

Not speed.

Not perfection.

Reliability.

If the first 90 days are about becoming safe enough to function, the first year is about becoming steady enough to grow. It is where the profession begins to move from something you are learning into something you are becoming.

And that transition matters.

Because a pharmacy career is not built in the classroom, and it is not built in orientation. It is built in the daily practice of showing up, paying attention, asking better questions, learning from what happens, and choosing accuracy again and again.

That is how confidence becomes earned.

That is how judgment becomes stronger.

That is how a new pharmacist becomes a professional.

45

GLOSSARY

About This Glossary

While not every one of these words appeared directly in this chapter, all terms marked with *(gl)* absolutely do. Since you're getting familiar with the world of a **Pharmacist**, this glossary will help you start speaking its language. Each word is part of the rhythm, tools, and teamwork that make this role come alive.

If you're serious about exploring a future in this field, give yourself a big jump by learning these terms now. They're more than vocabulary — they're the shorthand of care, the language of alignment, and the bridge between curiosity and confidence.

GLOSSARY — **Pharmacist**

ADC (Automated Dispensing Cabinet): Secure medication storage and dispensing unit used throughout hospitals to improve accuracy and access control.

Adherence: The extent to which a patient follows prescribed medication directions, including timing and dosage.

Adverse Drug Reaction (ADR): Harmful or unintended effect of a medication taken at normal doses.

Alaris Smart Pump: Infusion device used to deliver IV medications precisely, equipped with dose error reduction software.

Allergy Alert: A safety warning in pharmacy systems that prevents dispensing drugs known to cause reactions in a specific patient.

ASHP (American Society of Health-System Pharmacists): Professional organization representing pharmacists in hospitals and health systems.

Biosimilar: A biologic medical product highly similar to an already approved reference product, differing only in minor components.

Black Box Warning: The FDA's most serious medication warning, highlighting potential life-threatening risks.

Brand Name Drug: A medication sold under a trademarked name, patented by the manufacturer.

Capsule: Solid dosage form containing medication within a gelatin shell.

Central Pharmacy: The main hub within a hospital where pharmacists prepare, verify, and distribute medications.

Clinical Pharmacist: A pharmacist who provides direct patient care, optimizing medication therapy for safety and efficacy.

Compounding: The art of preparing customized medications to meet specific patient needs not covered by commercial products.

Controlled Substance: Drug regulated by the DEA due to potential for abuse or dependence.

DEA Schedule: Classification system for controlled substances (I–V) based on medical use and abuse potential.

Dispense: The act of preparing and providing medications to patients as authorized by a prescription.

Diverted Medication: Medication obtained or used outside its intended legal or clinical channel.

Drug Library Guardrails: Safety software within smart pumps that prevent incorrect dosing during infusion.

Drug Utilization Review (DUR): Process evaluating prescription orders for potential errors, interactions, or duplications.

EMR (Electronic Medical Record): Digital chart containing patient medical and medication history used by providers.

Formulary: A list of medications approved for use within a specific healthcare organization.

Generic Drug: Medication equivalent in active ingredients and dosage to a brand-name product but sold under its chemical name.

High-Alert Medication: Drug that carries a heightened risk of causing harm if used incorrectly.

IV Room: Sterile preparation area for intravenous medications following USP <797> standards.

ISMP (Institute for Safe Medication Practices): Organization dedicated to medication safety and error prevention.

LASA (Look-Alike/Sound-Alike): Medications with similar names or packaging that can lead to errors.

Medication Error: Any preventable event leading to inappropriate medication use or patient harm.

Medication Reconciliation: Process of ensuring an accurate medication list during transitions of care.

MME (Morphine Milligram Equivalent): Standard measure to compare opioid doses and assess risk.

Naloxone: Medication used to reverse opioid overdose.

NDC (National Drug Code): Unique identifier for every medication sold in the U.S.

Opioid Stewardship: Systematic approach to ensuring safe and appropriate opioid prescribing and monitoring.

Order Verification: Pharmacist process of reviewing prescriptions for accuracy, dose, and interactions before dispensing.

Over-the-Counter (OTC): Medications available without a prescription.

Par Level: Minimum quantity of a medication that must be stocked to meet patient care demands.

Patient Counseling: Pharmacist-provided education to patients about proper medication use and potential side effects.

PCA (Patient-Controlled Analgesia): Pump allowing patients to self-administer pain medication within preset safety limits.

Pharmacokinetics: Study of how a drug is absorbed, distributed, metabolized, and eliminated by the body.

Pharmacodynamics: Study of how drugs affect the body's systems and produce their effects.

Pharmacogenomics: Field studying how genes influence individual responses to drugs.

Pharmacy Informatics: Integration of technology and data analytics in managing medication systems.

PGY1 / PGY2: Postgraduate Year One and Two pharmacy residencies providing advanced clinical training.

Polypharmacy: Concurrent use of multiple medications by a single patient, often increasing risk of adverse effects.

Pyxis: Common brand of ADC used in hospital medication management.

Reconstitution: Process of mixing a powdered drug with a liquid for administration.

Reverse Distributor: Licensed facility that handles the return and disposal of expired or unused medications.

Route of Administration: The path by which a drug enters the body (oral, IV, IM, topical, etc.).

Therapeutic Duplication: Two or more drugs from the same class prescribed unnecessarily.

Therapeutic Index: Ratio between a drug's effective and toxic dose; narrow indexes require close monitoring.

Therapeutic Substitution: Replacing a prescribed drug with a chemically different but therapeutically equivalent medication.

Trough Level: Lowest concentration of a drug in the bloodstream before the next dose; used to guide dosing of certain antibiotics.

USP (United States Pharmacopeia): Organization establishing standards for medication quality, strength, and purity.

Vancomycin: Common IV antibiotic monitored for trough levels to prevent toxicity.

VTE Prophylaxis: Preventive measures, often involving medication, to reduce risk of blood clots.

. . .

Why This Matters

Learning the vocabulary of pharmacy is the first step toward understanding how safety, precision, and compassion intersect. Every one of these terms connects to a moment where a patient's outcome depends on clarity and care. If you're serious about exploring a career as a pharmacist, start here — mastering the language that saves lives.

46

ALSO BY MASON MAISON™

What Color Are Your Scrubs?

A Career Guide for Healthcare Professionals Seeking Alignment, Purpose, and Long-Term Fit

A foundational framework for understanding how healthcare careers actually feel—not just what they look like on paper. Designed to help readers make more informed, alignment-driven decisions before committing to a path.

The ScrubTales™ **Series**

Real-World Career Guides That Tell the Truth About Healthcare Roles

Each title in the ScrubTales™ series provides a detailed, experience-based look at a specific healthcare career, including Day in the Life narratives, decision frameworks, financial realities, and long-term career pathways.

Current Titles Include:

• **ScrubTales™: Nurse Practitioner**

A Real-World Career Guide That Tells the Truth About Advanced Practice, Autonomy, and Clinical Responsibility

- **ScrubTales™: Physician Assistant**

A Real-World Career Guide That Tells the Truth About Flexibility, Scope of Practice, and Team-Based Care

- **ScrubTales™: Registered Nurse**

A Real-World Career Guide That Tells the Truth About the Demands and Tradeoffs of Nursing

- **ScrubTales™: Surgical Technologist**

A Real-World Career Guide That Tells the Truth About the Operating Room and Surgical Teamwork

- **ScrubTales™: Diagnostic Medical Sonographer**

A Real-World Career Guide That Tells the Truth About Imaging, Precision, and Patient Interaction

- **ScrubTales™: Respiratory Therapist**

A Real-World Career Guide That Tells the Truth About Critical Care, Breathing Support, and Patient Stability

- **ScrubTales™: Clinical Pharmacist**

A Real-World Career Guide That Tells the Truth About Medication Management, Clinical Decision-Making, and System-Level Impact

- **ScrubTales™: Radiologic Technologist**

A Real-World Career Guide That Tells the Truth About Imaging Technology, Workflow, and Patient Care

- **ScrubTales™: Physical Therapist**

A Real-World Career Guide That Tells the Truth About Recovery, Movement, and Long-Term Patient Progress

- **ScrubTales™: Medical Laboratory Scientist**

A Real-World Career Guide That Tells the Truth About Diagnostics, Data, and Behind-the-Scenes Medicine

Coming Soon

Additional ScrubTales™ titles will continue expanding across healthcare careers, including:

- Licensed Practical Nurse (LPN)
- Medical Assistant

- Occupational Therapist
- Dental Assistant
- Medical & Health Services Manager
- Physical Therapist Assistant
- Speech-Language Pathologist
- Medical Records Specialist
- Home Health & Personal Care Aide
- Certified Nursing Assistant (CNA)

Explore More

Mason Maison™ Publishing focuses on alignment-first career guidance for healthcare professionals—helping individuals understand not just how to enter a field, but how to stay, grow, and thrive within it.

47

ABOUT THE AUTHOR

Mason Preddy is a healthcare workforce strategist, former executive recruiter, and the founder of Mason Maison™ Publishing. His work sits at the intersection of career decision-making, workforce alignment, and the real-world experience of working in healthcare—an area he has spent more than two decades studying, shaping, and influencing.

Before becoming an author and publisher, Mason built his career inside the healthcare recruitment and talent strategy space, where he worked closely with hospitals, health systems, and physician groups across the country. He served on the Board of Directors for the National Association of Health Care Recruiters (NAHCR), including as Treasurer, and played a role in advancing industry standards and certification efforts during a critical period of growth in healthcare talent acquisition.

Earlier in his career, Mason served as Director of the Healthcare Practice at TMP Worldwide, the recruitment advertising firm widely known for creating Monster.com. In that role, he worked with major healthcare organizations on national recruitment strategy, employer branding, and workforce positioning. He later continued that work with Bernard Hodes Group, part of Omnicom, where he focused exclusively on healthcare clients, including large hospital systems in highly competitive markets.

Throughout his career, Mason has worked behind the scenes in one of the most important—but least understood—areas of healthcare: how people enter, move through, and ultimately experience their careers in the field. He has seen firsthand how decisions made early—often with limited information—can shape not only careers, but lives.

That perspective became the foundation for his writing.

Mason is the author of *What Color Are Your Scrubs?*, a career framework designed to help individuals understand not just what healthcare jobs exist, but how those roles actually feel on a daily basis. Rather than focusing solely on job descriptions, salaries, and educational pathways, his work centers on alignment—how personality, environment, expectations, and lived experience intersect to determine long-term career sustainability.

From that foundation, the *ScrubTales*™ series was created.

Each book in the series is designed to go beyond surface-level career guidance and instead provide a real-world, experience-based look at healthcare roles—what they demand, what they offer, and how they fit different types of individuals. Through detailed Day in the Life narratives, structured frameworks, and practical insights, the series aims to give readers a level of clarity that is rarely available before entering the field.

Mason's approach is rooted in a simple but often overlooked idea:

People do not burn out from caring.

They burn out from working in roles that do not fit who they are.

This belief has shaped not only his writing, but his broader body of work.

In addition to his publishing efforts, Mason is the creator of HIRE Intelligence™, a platform focused on helping healthcare professionals understand how they are evaluated, hired, and positioned within organizations. Drawing on more than 25 years of experience in recruiting and leadership hiring, his work provides insight into the hidden dynamics of healthcare careers—from resumes and interviews to long-term advancement and leadership positioning.

He is also the founder of SaplingOak™, a healthcare workforce strategy initiative focused on physician, advanced practice provider, and executive-level recruitment and alignment. His work in this space continues to influence how organizations think about talent, retention, and long-term workforce sustainability.

Across all of his work—books, platforms, and consulting—Mason's focus remains consistent:

Helping people make better career decisions before they commit to paths that may not fit them.

His writing is known for combining real-world experience with practical clarity—avoiding both idealized portrayals and unnecessary negativity. Instead, he focuses on giving readers an honest, usable understanding of what different roles require and how those roles align with different types of individuals.

Mason believes that better-informed decisions lead to more sustainable careers, stronger healthcare systems, and ultimately better patient outcomes.

Because when people are aligned with their work, everything works better.

AFTERWORD

Afterword: Pharmacist

Thank you for allowing me to walk beside you as you explored the possibilities of becoming a pharmacist. I hope you leave with a clearer sense of the work, the heart, and the hope behind every prescription. The profession is waiting for curious minds and steady hands like yours—because the future of care depends on them.

Pharmacy shows what happens when precision meets compassion. It's the science that sustains life and the humanity that gives it meaning. Accuracy isn't cold—it's care, delivered with intention.

Every pharmacist begins in the classroom—building knowledge, discipline, and confidence long before the first patient encounter. That education isn't just preparation; it's the foundation of safe, exceptional care.

And if you discover that pharmacy isn't your forever fit, take that as progress—not disappointment. Exploring healthcare is about uncovering where your strengths, values, and energy belong. Alignment grows through reflection, honesty, and the courage to begin again. My hope for you is simple: **do whatever makes you thrive.** And if it isn't this—if pharmacy isn't the space where your spark feels at home—**life is too short not to find the career that will make you thrive.**

Continue exploring the *What Color Are Your Scrubs?* book series, designed to help you discover where your heart and skills align. The flagship book, *What Color Are Your Scrubs?*, takes a deeper dive into purpose, burnout, and alignment across every corner of the profession. Take the **SCRUB*fit*™ Healthcare Career Assessment**, powered by the **Alignment Intelligence Model**—a proprietary blend of personality science, purpose values, and behavioral fit—to match you with the roles where you're most likely to thrive.

Every resource I've built exists to help you move forward with clarity, confidence, and direction as you design the career that truly fits you.

Wherever you serve, lead with clarity, act with compassion, and remember—the heart of healthcare will always need hands like yours. I wish you lots of continued success.

Goodbye for now,

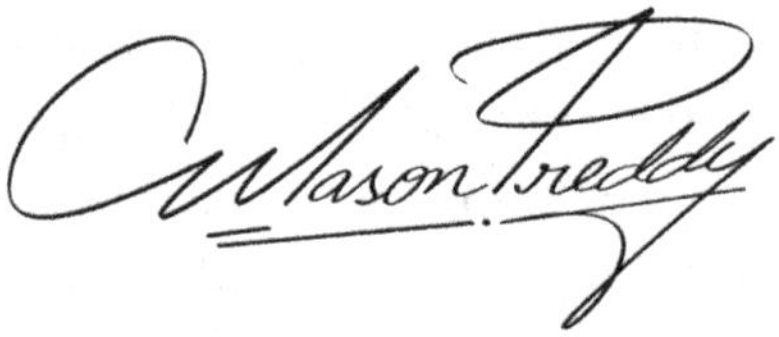

Made in the USA
Monee, IL
05 November 2026

67911939R00154